REIKI

Guided Meditation for Unblocking,
Developing and Balancing Your Psychic Empath
Abilities and Positive Energy

(A Self-healing & Meditation Guide to
Kickstart Aura Cleansing)

Sarah Koda

Published by Rob Miles

Sarah Koda

All Rights Reserved

Reiki: Guided Meditation for Unblocking, Developing and Balancing Your Psychic Empath Abilities and Positive Energy (A Self-healing & Meditation Guide to Kickstart Aura Cleansing)

ISBN 978-1-989990-34-6

All rights reserved. No part of this guide may be reproduced in any form without permission in writing from the publisher except in the case of brief quotations embodied in critical articles or reviews.

Legal & Disclaimer

The information contained in this book is not designed to replace or take the place of any form of medicine or professional medical advice. The information in this book has been provided for educational and entertainment purposes only.

The information contained in this book has been compiled from sources deemed reliable, and it is accurate to the best of the Author's knowledge; however, the Author cannot guarantee its accuracy and validity and cannot be held liable for any errors or omissions. Changes are periodically made to this book. You must consult your doctor or get professional medical advice before using any of the suggested remedies, techniques, or information in this book.

Upon using the information contained in this book, you agree to hold harmless the Author from and against any damages, costs, and expenses, including any legal fees potentially resulting from the application of any of the information provided by this guide. This disclaimer applies to any damages or injury caused by the use and application, whether directly or indirectly, of any advice or information presented, whether for breach of contract, tort, negligence, personal injury, criminal intent, or under any other cause of action.

You agree to accept all risks of using the information presented inside this book. You need to consult a professional medical practitioner in order to ensure you are both able and healthy enough to participate in this program.

Table of Contents

INTRODUCTION 1

CHAPTER 1: WHAT IS ENERGY HEALING? 3

CHAPTER 2: REIKI PRINCIPLES AND SYMBOLS 10

CHAPTER 3: WHAT YOU SHOULD KNOW ABOUT REIKI AS A BEGINNER 20

CHAPTER 4: BENEFITS OF REIKI 38

CHAPTER 5: CRYSTALS AND MEDITATION FOR THE THIRD EYE 47

CHAPTER 6: REIKI AND YOUR CHAKRA 55

CHAPTER 7: HOW TO BECOME A REIKI CHANNEL 60

CHAPTER 8: THE BENEFITS OF REIKI HEALING 72

CHAPTER 9: CHAKRAS AND THE AURA 78

CHAPTER 10: USING REIKI WITH OTHERS 93

CHAPTER 11: THE SEVEN CHAKRAS................................. 100

CHAPTER 12: FORGIVENESS.. 106

CHAPTER 13: HOW CAN YOU EXPERIENCE MAGNIFICENCE? 112

CHAPTER 14: IMPROVE YOUR LIFE WITH REIKI 123

CHAPTER 15: WHAT TO EXPECT FROM A REIKI SESSION 128

CHAPTER 16: REIKI HEALING AND SELF-HEALING........... 132

CHAPTER 17: REIKI AND ALTERNATIVE THERAPEUTIC DISCIPLINES 150

CHAPTER 18: BLACK TOURMALINE AND REIKI 161

CHAPTER 19: REIKI BASICS 170

CHAPTER 20: USING CRYSTALS IN REIKI 186

CONCLUSION 193

Introduction

The person being healed, wherein we will refer to as Customers, may encounter a secret government of unwinding during a Reiki session. They may likewise feel warm, tingly, lethargic, or revived. Reiki gives off an impression of being commonly protected, and no genuine symptoms have been accounted for.

No unique foundation or accreditations are expected to get preparing. Be that as it may, Reiki must be gained from an accomplished instructor or a Master; it can't act naturally educated. The particular strategies educated can shift significantly. Preparing in conventional Reiki has three degrees or levels, each concentrating on an alternate part of the training. Every degree incorporates at least one inception. Additionally, these are called attunements or strengthening influences. Getting inception is accepted to enact the capacity to get to Reiki vitality.

There are a lot of books regarding this matter available, thanks again for picking this one! Each exertion was made to guarantee it is loaded with however much helpful data as could be expected!

Chapter 1: What Is Energy Healing?

The idea of energy healing is a very broad subject, as there are multiple methods that can be used to accomplish the same goal. The linked goal between all of these practices is to realign the body's natural energy fields in order to restore health and wellness. That too sounds pretty broad, so let's explore that for a minute by thinking about why we would need to do this in the first place.

What we know is that the body is made up of energy. The atoms and molecules that make us up can be pared down to sets of positive and negative particles that interact with each other. In nature, energy prefers to flow a certain way, and if anything is done to disturb that interaction, it creates a chain reaction wave that offsets energy elsewhere. Now, this can apply to one organ in the body, our entire beings, and the way that we interact with the world.

The idea of energy can be a tough concept to grasp, as it cannot be tangibly seen, at least not to the average person. Everything in the universe is simply the energy we talked about before. When broken down, there are only positive and negative charges. All living things, human and animal alike, have developed brains that sort out the waves of energy that are perceived in the environment and make sense of them.

Our five senses are available to sense energy waves, which are then computed in the brain to develop a sight, smell, taste, sound or feeling that will be associated with this energy. For example, sitting under a pine tree gives us the sense of branches and leaves, and the smell of pine.

Energy healing has been around for ages and is believed to have originated somewhere in the Eastern region, in countries like India and Nepal. The idea that the universe is made up of energy was well known throughout the ancient cultures of every civilization, including

Native Americans in the United States, half way across the world from India.

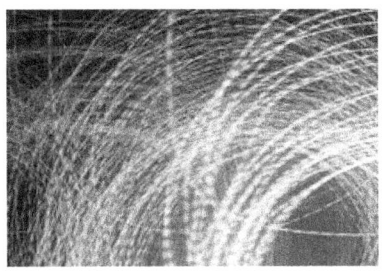

Ascivilization dragged on, people became less in-tune with this fact, often turning to pharmaceutical medications to soothe what ailed them, whether a physical problem like arthritis or an emotional issue like depression. As a whole, humans were more willing to go with the efforts of modern medicine, rather than realigning a somewhat intangible energy field that could solve all of their problems.

Sure, the idea of the world being created by an intangible energy may seem like hocus pocus, but then we must also consider the workings of one of the greatest minds in history, that of Albert

Einstein. His famous theories were based on the fact that the universe is just energy, and there is a specific order to it. Everything is interconnected because ultimately, we are all a part of the same energy field.

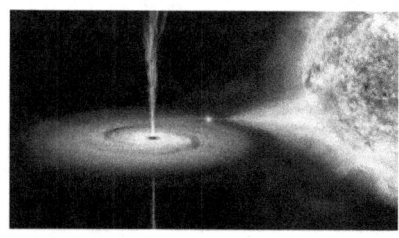

Even more recently, Dr. Wilhelm Reich discovered that imbalanced energy within the confines of the body caused disease and distress, and fixing the energy would cure the ailment. This is the direction we would like to discuss more, as physical and emotional ailments are at the center of our health and well-being.

Luckily, there are groups of practitioners in existence that are still knowledgeable about universal energy and how it affects the body. These are the people who are most in-tune with the body today. The good news is, these ideas are also backed by science.

For centuries, practitioners spoke of a 'third eye.' This invisible eye was something everyone had, and it was the connection between the body in the flesh and its spiritual being. In pictures, it is depicted as a literal eye located just above and between our eyes. While not clearly visible to the naked eye, it was thought to be the eye that saw the most and was responsible for our emotional response to the world. Myths tell of supernatural powers being activated as the third eye awakens. If activated, we are able to see the future, tap into the full potential of our intuition, and be a step ahead of our counterparts.

The third eye acts as a sixth sense, allowing us to see above and beyond, including into different realms and universes. Instead of detecting sights and smells, your third eye detects patterns across your life. It can show you patterns of how you react in certain situations, things you gravitate toward, positive and

negative, and when listened to, can be a guiding force to set you in the right direction. For some people, tapping into their sixth sense gives them the ability to see
auras or the physical manifestation of energy surrounding a person. A body will emit a glow of varying varieties of color, which can usually be related to their personality and mood. We all emit these auras, but only a select few can actually see them.

Modern science has mapped the brain and found that this third eye actually exists. It does not work like a typical eye, in fact, it is responsible for much more. The pineal gland, which is centered in the middle of the brain, and, if our skulls were see-through, would be seen right on the forehead, as the mystical third eye was once imagined.

While the tiny gland remains a mystery, it is responsible for releasing the hormone melatonin, which regulates your circadian sleep and wake rhythms. This hormone is key to overall function and vitality in life, and we literally cannot live without it. The full potential of this pea-sized gland still remains to be discovered, and we will anxiously await those results.

Lots of things can set off an energy imbalance, including stress from the environment, inner turmoil and even physical problems like the decline in health. The goal of any type of energy healing is to offset this energy imbalance where it lives so that the body and spirit may come back to center, where it functions at its best.

The practices that will be discussed in the following chapters are just a few of the many offshoots of practices that involve energy healing. It is important that you experiment will have any option you come across, as everyone is a little bit different, and one method may click with you more than another, depending on what your needs are. Pay attention to your energy and mood while doing any given practice to determine if carrying on is right for you.

Chapter 2: Reiki Principles And Symbols

Before you can begin any form of Reiki healing you must know the basic components of the system of healing that Reiki uses. There are five basic elements that are utilized whether you are healing yourself or another. Keeping this list handy will ensure that you are always prepared to give or receive Reiki healing.

Attunements: Also known as initiations when used in Reiki healing this is known as being in tune with the energy. Being in tune with Reiki energy guarantees that you will be able to channel the energy properly.

Hand positions: These are important in Reiki healing and involve knowing where to put your hands during the healing. They can be split into two forms, treating yourself and treating others.

Meditation: The easiest way to focus with the Ki in the body and preform Reiki healing is to meditate or focus on the energy within yourself.

Symbols: Use the symbols of Reiki were needed and use the sound their name makes as a mantra when you need to connect with the energy.

Reiki Principles: There are give basic principles to Reiki healing and they should be used daily as a source of encouragement and during meditation before you heal yourself or another.

Now knowing this basic list and always keeping it handy in your mind, or even in a print off, we need to look at some of the concepts more closely. The first and most important arc the five principles of Reiki:

Principle 1*:* For today, I will not be angry I will focus on goodwill

When you have a focus of anger or upset whether it be at yourself, your loved ones or what is going on in the world you create blockages in your energy. It is the biggest and most complex of the inner demons we all battle with. Reiki is the right tool to remove those blockages caused by anger. These pools can be accumulated over a short period of long period and still be removed. While Reiki can remove the pools it cannot remove the source of anger. Letting go of your anger will bring peace into your mind and energy.

Principle 2: For today, I will not worry

Like anger, worry causes blocks, but worry tends to stem more from future events. The more worrying that we keep in our minds, the more pools and blockages it can cause. Where anger needs a focused Reiki healing to undo, worry needs the energy to be spread throughout the entirety of the body and mind. When you let go of things and stop worrying you bring healing to your body.

Principle 3: For today, I will be grateful

Be grateful starting with your heart and spreading throughout your entire body. Small things count, such as smiling at someone, offering kind words, showing gratitude and giving thanks. These small things all count and when you are thankful you bring joy to your soul.

Principle 4: For today, I will do my work with truth

This means to support yourself and your family in a way that does not bring harm to other living beings. Earn a living, but do so in a respectable way, make sure your life is lived with honor. Working truthfully will bring love to the will of mind and body.

Principle 5: For today, I will be kind to anything that lives.

Bring honor to your family, by being kind. Show kindness to all things great and small be they human, animal or plant. By being kind you bring more love into the will of the mind and body.

The next important tool in Reiki is knowing the symbols, they are considered sacred and some are not revealed until your second or third level of mastery. For the purposes of this book, as a beginner to Reiki there are just a few basic ones to know, and use as mantra.

ChoKuRay

Said: choh

koo

ray

Also called: "The symbol of Force"

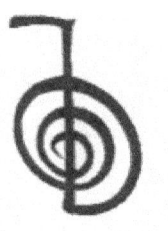

Means: Deity and mortal being coming together

This symbol is most commonly employed to directly increase the power of Reiki it will draw energy from around the healer and will go where you focus it. To use it you will make the sign over yourself or the person you are healing and silently say the word Cho Ku Rei 3 times.

This symbol is one that can be employed anytime for anything. Including:

Emergency treatments

Treatments done at once with little preparation

To clean an area of negative energy

For protection of the spirit

To cleanse food, drinks, medicine and herbs of negative energy.

At the hospital for healing

To give more power to other symbols

To seal in healing energy that has been placed for treatment.
SeiHeiKi
Said: say
hay
key
Also called: The symbol of the mind and feeling

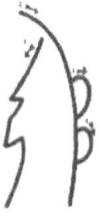

Meaning: The opener of the universe
This symbol is most commonly employed in healing that involves cerebral or sentimental problems. It is good to calm the mind and is also best used for:
Protection against physic attack
Mental cleansing
During meditations
For balancing both sides of the brain

To aid in overcoming addictions
Healing trauma
Aligning the upper chakras
Removing negative energy
HonShaZeShoNen
Said: Hanh
shah
zay
show
nen
Also called: The Space Symbol

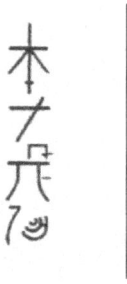

Meaning: The deity within me greets you
This symbol is employed in distance Reiki healing. You will draw and use it when you wish to send healing energy to anyone that isn't directly in a room with you.
TamAraSha

Said: Tam
ara
sha
Also called: The Harmony Symbol

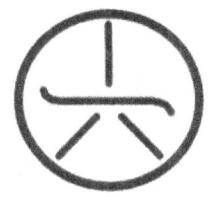

This symbol is employed to bring balance and harmony to the body and soul and will also strengthen Reiki energy being used to bring down a blockage. It is used commonly for:

Grounding energy

Balancing energy

Unblocking energy especially, at chakra centers.

Used over painful areas to reduce or completely do away with the pain.

The final item from the list that is used overall is attunement. In general a deep attunement can only be done for you by a Reiki Master, so if you plan on a full attunement or going deeper with your Reiki practices than a beginner level you should consider finding a Master who can attune you. However, there are basic steps that you can do as a beginner to attune yourself.

Step 1: Sit in a place that has no distractions, soft music can be played and prepare yourself as if preparing for meditation. Center yourself.

Step 2: With your right hand draw the symbols of ChoKuRay, SeiHeiKi and TamAraSha on your forehead.

Step 3: Visualize your chakra's and the energy that radiates from them. Follow that flow outward and through your body and aura. As you visualize chant the three symbols, names quietly three times.

Step 4: Lightly touch your forehead again, the third eye and visualize the constant flow of energy, balance and how you can share that energy with others to heal them or heal yourself.

Once you feel you have centered yourself enough and have a firm grasp on your own inner Ki, you are attuned on a basic level and can preform the beginners Reiki healing that is in the next chapters.

Chapter 3: What You Should Know About Reiki As A Beginner

The term "Reiki" simply means the flow of miraculous sign and energy from the atmosphere. It of healing energy.

What is Reiki?

Reiki is a Japanese practice with a designation that means "universal life energy." It's a method based on the concept that the practitioner can facilitate the flow and smooth transmission of the customer's own spiritual energy through contact or proximity. In the late 1930s, Mrs.

Hawayo Takata brought Reiki largely to the west from Japan. Over time, Takata passed on her knowledge to others, and the technique spread throughout the west.

The physician softly touches the patient with both hands in particular positions during a Reiki session or hold their hands above the patient slightly. Typically, Reiki sessions last about an hour. The practitioner places his or her hands during the session, on or over the patient's body in up to 15 distinct traditional hand positions, holding each position for two to five minutes at a moment. The therapy is totally non-invasive and does not require any manipulation of tissue or painful pressure.

How Does it Work?

People who practice Reiki know that there are blocked energy pathways that exemplify pain and disease in the body. The objective of Reiki treatments is to increase energy flow through these blocked or troubled pathways, this reduces pain and increases the natural capacity of the body to battle disease and cure itself. Reiki can assist decrease pain associated with the development of the disease in cancer patients. It can also decrease some of the unpleasant symptoms frequently experienced by patients during cancer therapy such as depression, lack of strength, and vomiting. In addition, Reiki can also enhance the emotional health and perspective of the patient, which may enhance the capacity and readiness of the patient to follow the directions of the physician and stick to therapy protocols.

It is said that Reiki involves transferring universal energy from the palms of the practitioner to their patient. Energy healing has been used in different forms for millennia. Advocates argue that it operates with the body's energy fields. A 2007 study reveals that at least once in the past

years, 1 million plus adolescents in the United States (U.S.) attempted Reiki or comparable therapy. It is thought that more than 60 hospitals give patients Reiki services.

Reiki Attunement, What Is It?

The method through which an individual gets the capacity to give Reiki treatments is Reiki attunement. During the Reiki class, the attunement is administered by the Reiki Master. During the attunement, The Reiki Master touches the head, hands, and shoulders and of the person and uses one or more unique relaxation techniques. Attunement energies will flow into the person through the Reiki Master. The Higher Power guides these unique energies and makes changes in the energy pathways of the learners and connects the student to Reiki's source. Since the Higher Power guides the energetic aspect of the tuning, it adjusts for each student to be precisely correct. Some people feel warm in their hands during the tuning, others may see colors or have spiritual beings visions. However, for the tuning to have worked, it is not essential to have an inner experience. Most of it just feels more relaxed.

You're Considering Learning Reiki?

Reiki is a very easy learning method and is not dependent on having any previous experience with healing, meditation or any other type of practice. More than a million individuals from all walks of life have discovered it effectively, the young as well as old. More reason why learning it is so simple is that it's learned without been pre-trained. The capacity to do Reiki is simply transmitted from the teacher through a mechanism called an attunement during a Reiki class to the student. Immediately one receives an attunement; they possess the ability to do Reiki after which whenever one places their hands on themselves or someone else to do Reiki, the healing energy automatically will begin flowing.

Starting A Reiki Practice

Whether you're just beginning a Reiki practice to provide Reiki healing for customers or patients in need or you're planning to give Reiki training to teach others how to deliver Reiki treatments, Starting a Reiki company enables you to give a bigger amount of individuals this unique therapy. It may also be a source of income to start a Reiki practice – there is increasing demand for this secure and efficient strategy to Reiki healing.

Just like opening up any other form of company, starting the Reiki practice needs foresight and planning. Once you understand how to begin a Reiki company, healing typically begins dramatically.

Planning to Start Reiki Business

You're going to want to know everything about Reiki first and then find a Reiki Master Teacher to study with. Then you will finish training classes on Reiki, practicing at home and on yourself and potentially family or friends. Before you start on your own, it is vital that you get well-rounded schooling in Reiki. It is essential for you to be comfortable with the Reiki energy before providing Reiki services to others.

Where To Practice

Look for a place to treat Reiki. Some districts enable Reiki professionals from their own homes to function. You might prefer to lease a room, maybe share a room with a surgeon, health therapist or massage therapist. Whether you're planning to provide Reiki healing at home or in a leased firm room, the facility needs to provide your customers with privacy and convenience.

Get a Reiki Table

Invest in a nice table for bodywork. If you are unable to afford a fresh one, we're in a digital globe, a search on the internet for quality would do or contact local massage schools for some Reiki tables suggestions that practitioners discovered to be comfortable, portable, and low-cost.

Gain Experience and Build Your Client Base
Develop a client base and acquire expertise by contracting or volunteering in hospitals, nursing homes, hospices, and other facilities where patients may benefit from Reiki medicines. are there any assisting organizations that might profit from your moment with Reiki or volunteering? A position dear to your heart's cause?

Spread the Word
Let others understand you're beginning a practice of Reiki. Ask friends, family and customers or patients with whom you have worked to write testimonials for you to publish or show as printed reviews on your website. Recommendations are always better than advertising that is paid.

Your Reiki Treatments

Treat every client of Reiki as a precious person. It should be slow, meticulous and professional for Reiki treatments. The meeting has everything to do with the client. You are there as a Reiki practitioner to promote a relaxing and well-being atmosphere for your customers. As an additional side advantage to you, Observe up at the end of the session with each client to ensure that the healing or relaxation method continues after the end of the Reiki session and to offer any help to questions they may have. The longer you exercise Reiki and experience its advantages, the more you will certainly be motivated to continue your Reiki education. To learn more about Reiki techniques or brush up on your current Reiki abilities, attend Reiki training classes. It's simple to start a Reiki exercise once all the details are known. Finding a regular exercise that takes you away from ' day to day ' is so essential to remind you that it's all right. ' said by Ian Tucker in Your Simple Path – Find happiness in every step.

The quote describes what Reiki is – the touch of healing. To enhance one's health and quality of life is a life force energy. In its recovery, it has a spiritual element. For ' Higher Power, ' ' Rei ' is
the Japanese term and ' ki ' is the energy of life force. That is to say, Reiki is an ' energy of life force spiritually guided. '

Time Taken while learning Reiki

On a weekend, a starting Reiki class is taught. The class may last for one or two days. I consider at least six to seven hours for the minimum moment needed. Together with the attunement, it's essential to show the student how to treat and also how to exercise treatment in the environment.

Putting Reiki in perspective

Reiki is an interaction of a person individually. It is unlikely that anyone who does not believe the therapy will experience any benefit of it. One of Reiki's main principles is that it would not cause damage because it is applied without tampering or force but only using a light touch, for individuals with pain, restricted mobility, or extreme weakness, it is recommended.

About Reiki Hand Positions – the Basics

Going in for your first therapy, these are the positions that you can usually expect to use because they are typical of most therapy sessions. Every other position is designed to balance the energies in that region and remove stuck energies so you can start relaxing, Reduce stress and allow your body to rest and heal and work better. If you need special attention to be given to one region, let your physician know. Your physician will often be able to detect regions within the hand positions that need additional attention that may not even have been revealed to you.

Positions of Hand During Reiki Application

In Reiki, there are basic typical and basic hand positions taught in Reiki certification classes that are used to encourage energy distribution and healing to different fields of the body. During a Reiki therapy, more time may be spent on one region than another depending on your specific health problem. This article, commonly speaking, highlights the fundamental Reiki hand positions. And/or during a session, some of the hand positions may be omitted in a distinct order. Depending on your individual requirements, variations can also be made on these roles.

Expectation During Treatment With Reiki

A customer rests comfortably on a massage table during a Reiki session or is sometimes sitting on a chair. There is no tissue manipulation occurring in massage or bodywork, but only a very gentle pressure of the hand. Unlike massage treatment, during a Reiki session, you are always completely clothed. The session generally takes place in silence with a relatively no conversation, unless you want to tell your practitioner something, then it's essential that you do it quickly. Your Reiki practitioner can play relaxing background music or sounds of nature. If you're awkward or comfortable, or the music is distracting, for instance, or you prefer to skip some Reiki hand position, just let your physician know before or during your session.

The Reiki "Touch"

Reiki is conducted either with very gentle, static pressure from the practitioner's hands on traditional hand-positioned fields, or with a few inches above your body with their hands. In either case, Reiki works almost as well, so if you prefer the hovering method over being touched directly, let your practitioner know before the session begins. During a Reiki session, sensitive or private regions will never be affected. Even if in a delicate or private region you have a health problem, it is against the Code of Ethics of a Reiki Professional Practitioner to physically touch personal or sensual regions. Your Reiki practitioner wants you to feel refreshed and be comfortable as possible while enjoying this timeless Japanese energy technique work for stress reduction, relaxation, and well-being.

Some of the most popular general hand positions in the Reiki session that you could encounter:

Position A

Palms are put on your forehead lightly and/or the fingers of the practitioner may cup your eyes softly.

Position B

The physician could also put his hands on the edges of your temples and face soothingly.

Position C

The practitioner's hands may cradle your head as his or her hands rest on the table.

Position D

Reiki can be provided softly to your jawline or throat region.

Position E

Either of the practitioner's hand might well swing or be positioned near your throat or above your collarbone, while your other hand may swing or be positioned above your chakra core which is around your heart region.

Position F

Hands can be softly put on your pelvic area.

Position G

The physician can put his hands on your solar plexus or mid-abdomen

Position H

The practitioner can put his hands on your lower middle abdomen a few inches below your navel.

Position I

A physician may preferably give Reiki to your knees and/or wrists or feet. If the physician feels they can benefit you, these are alternative positions. Or they can just move on to your back's side positions.

Position J

The physician may ask you to turn on your belly with your head in a face cradle or softly resting on one side if you are on a massage table. The hands of the practitioner are softly put and rested on your shoulder blade region.

Position K

Hands are shifted below your shoulder blades or the middle back area of the body.

Position L

The physician moves his hands to apply gentle pressure on your lower back with soft hand placement.

Once all the fundamental positions and/or variants are covered and energies are lifted or balanced, the physician can move his hands over your body in a sweeping movement to clean your energy field from any remaining energy residue, Leaving you clean, feeling happy and strengthening your well-being path.

Afterward

Feel free to keep your body hydrated after your session for 24 hours and take some time after your session, even just a few minutes, to observe peace and quietness. Try to enable yourself to gain gratitude from your greater self for caring so eloquently for your body, mind, and spirit sometime after your workout or perhaps later in the evening before bed and to appreciate your enhanced state of well-being and peace.

Can I Treat Myself?

Yes, you could also treat yourself as well as others once you have got the attunement. This is one of Reiki's distinctive characteristics. I've heard Reiki can be performed from a distance to others.

How Is This Going To Work?

You are provided 3 Reiki symbols in Reiki II (Deeper Level). The attunement to Reiki II empowers these symbols. One of these symbols is for remote healing by using an image of the individual you want to send Reiki to or by writing the name of the individual on a piece of paper or simply thinking about the individual and activating the remote symbol, No matter where they are, you can send Reiki to them. They might be thousands of miles away, but that doesn't matter. The energy from Reiki is going to go to them and treat them. You can also send Reiki to disasters or global leaders, and they will also be aided by Reiki energy.

How many Reiki training levels are there?

There are four levels in Reiki's Usui / Tibetan scheme taught by the Center. These include the first, the second, the Advanced and the Master.

Can A Reiki Individual Be Earning A Living From It?

If you put your heart into it, coupled with teaching courses, you can create a Reiki practice that can generate a periodic revenue. This is a very satisfying way of earning a living.

Can One Be Licensed For Reiki Activity And Teaching?

At this moment, there is no government licensing programs. However, for Reiki educators, However, there are International Centers and Teachers Guidebook available from these Center, the Centers have a licensing program.

Does Reiki Treatment Cover Insurance?

Insurance companies are just beginning to recognize Reiki. Although not many of them cover Reiki treatments, there are some.

Can Nurses Nurses Or Yoga Teachers Take Reiki Courses?

Courses conducted by Reiki teachers' centers are endorsed to be offered to nurses, massage therapists and athletic trainers with adequate training and certificates.

Reiki Lineage

Reiki is a method that is continuously transferred from professor to student. If you have Reiki, then you will be part of a sequence of educators that will lead back to the Reiki system founder that you are practicing. The lineage, for example, is traced to Dr. Usui in the case of the Usui Reiki lineage.

Chapter 4: Benefits Of Reiki

Reiki has multiple benefits and uses, from supporting the health of the physical body to reaching the state of mental-emotional-spiritual balance. Through Reiki we will attract into our lives what we need at a particular time in order to be healthy, balanced and happy. However, we need to understand that Reiki is not a panacea and it will not make problems disappear; it is an „instrument" that helps us to overcome the obstacles and challenges of this existence easier, at all their Levels of manifestation if we PRACTICE EVERY DAY.

Reiki stimulates the immune system, supports the recovery of the body, stimulates the ability of the body to eliminate toxins, increases physical vitality and stamina, but it is by no means a quick healing method. With every Reiki seminar I highlight the fact that those who graduate the course and practice Reiki, do not have the right to declare themselves healers, even if they may have results with Reiki.

Although in the common language we are sometimes using the terms „patient", „therapy" and „healing" or we are making references by using actual medical situations, Reiki practitioners should be aware that they are using Universal energy in the „therapy", not their personal energy. Therefore, they cannot take credit for the results achieved; they are just pure channels for Reiki. This is the reason why I believe it is not moral to take credit for being „healers"; we are Reiki practitioners. After the Reiki initiation, the various energetic Levels of the body become balanced, the aura becomes brighter and has finer vibrations. This change of the aura can be confirmed by measuring devices that evaluate the energetic field; however, this change can also be felt by children or pets. Children, for instance, will be very happy to see a person who has just received their initiation; dogs may look at their owners, sniff them for a few seconds and then will want to stay in their aura. Children and animals have more „senses" and they will feel this transformation. It is natural since after the initiation older imbalances or information, or older illnesses/diseases which have an „imprint" in the energetic field are being eliminated and the vibrations of this field become finer. About devices measuring imbalances and/or the vibration of our energies: it was interesting when I underwent such a procedure, after I had performed an initiation the previous day.

The physician who performed this procedure noticed the brightness of the aura which was captured even at a cellular Level by the device.

Reiki stimulates the functions of the organism and accelerates the healing/recovery processes of the body. If for instance, in the case of a fracture, the cast is usually kept on for six weeks, when I used Reiki 30 minutes/day the result was a complete recovery of the bone structure in three weeks without traces of calcification. In the case of sprains and pulls the respective area will be energized to reduce pain and to stimulate the healing process of the affected tissue, after having received medical treatment.

After a surgery, when Reiki has been used for 20-30 minutes daily, the wound healed more quickly and the tissue recovered without infection. A positive influence on healing and recovery was achieved through Reiki. I used Reiki for cuts, grazes and burns without placing the hand directly on the skin/wound, only from a 4-6 cm distance; the bleeding stopped faster and the skin healed in a shorter time.

Reiki does not produce some miracle through which the disease disappears, but it stimulates the immune system, therefore sustaining faster healing of viral infections, infections and allergies. I used to spend 3-4 days in bed with a viral infection; now I don't feel overwhelmed anymore and my recovery is quick, it may even take just a few hours. When others have colds and I am using Reiki on them they start sweating, they are feeling heat in the area where I am holding my hands on and after about 15-20 minutes they start feeling better. If the person already has a fever, which shows the body's defense mechanisms kicking in, I do not use Reiki on the head; I energize the spleen, the solar plexus, the umbilicus and the sole of the foot; this is how the heat is flowing from the head towards the limbs. A cold means the presence of the element Water, meaning „cold", fever being the element of Fire, therefore „heat"; the two have a tendency to balance each other out in order to achieve the state of health. This is why the body is reacting with a fever when we have accumulated cold.

Reiki acts on the cause of the health issue, freeing the body from symptoms in a natural way. So if we are feeling pain in a particular part of our bodies we can hold our hands directly on that area or we can look for the cause of the imbalance/problem in the physical body. We will notice how the pain will lessen, and often even disappear. If the condition requires other solutions, not just healing through energy, we should see a specialist. For instance, for pains caused by dental abscesses, we can use Reiki and we will feel how after 1-2 minutes of increased pulsations, the pain will be less intense. But it will not disappear entirely as dental treatment is required.

There were instances when I used Reiki on people with angina pectoris or mild heart attacks. The ambulance was called; in the meantime (5-10 minutes) the patient's condition had improved and the stabilizing/recovery process had begun. I will say this again, by using Reiki we have no right to declare ourselves healers, so please ask for medical treatment and do not ignore it. In situations like these, call the ambulance/physician, but help the patient with Reiki in the meantime. For hypertension, we energize the kidney area, the heart chakra and the renal pelvis, in the area opposite the umbilicus. Reiki also helps to balance the heart rate and gradually decrease (in about 3-6 months) the amount of medication for hypertension. However, the medicine dosage will only be changed by the treating physician, after a consultation.

Reiki makes it easier for the body to deal with the physical challenges during sports or strenuous activities. We can use Reiki on sore muscles after intense physical activity or a workout. If we go mountain climbing we can use Reiki directly on the area exhibiting cramps or on overstrained joints. To those suffering from rheumatic pain I recommend 30 minutes of Reiki daily and a proper diet.

Did you have a hard day? Are you feeling tired? I recommend daily self-energizing for those who have stressful jobs or are working with a lot of people. Reiki can be practiced anytime and anywhere, without being spectacular. This is how you can win back your energy even in a business meeting, without attracting attention. Reiki prevents burn-outs. Reiki helps eliminate fatigue and helps the organism recover. When driving and feeling tired, we can use Reiki on the heart chakra and the solar plexus. We will start noticing how we regain our attention and vigilance. When I was studying I used to apply Reiki before exams, instead of drinking coffee;

or when I had a thick head from the volume of information absorbed. I would spend 10-15 minutes with the palms on my head, on both cerebral hemispheres. This is how I was receiving clarification for my ideas.

Reiki helps eliminate toxic or harmful substances from the body, regardless of whether these come from foods, cigarettes, alcohol, the air, water or from invasive treatments like chemotherapy or radiotherapy. Even after your first Reiki initiation you will notice how your urine may have a different smell or that you may not be able to smoke like you used to. For the elimination of toxins Reiki will be applied on the affected area, on the liver and kidney area, in order to support these organs/areas of the body. Reiki can be used when someone has taken in more alcohol than the body is able to assimilate. If there are too many toxins stored in the body Reiki will not allow the use of that particular substance/food that caused the „saturation", for a while. There were instances when course participants have complained about how their habits were spoiled and they could no longer drink the same amount of coffee or alcohol, or that they could no longer smoke on an empty stomach. In the case of invasive therapies or investigations, when healthy cells or organs are also affected, Reiki can eliminate the toxic substances accumulated and will help the organism recover. For people suffering from constipation or hemorrhoids I use Reiki on the stomach area, the umbilical chakra and the root chakra, thus regulating the elimination of toxins and also helping them release selfishness.

Chapter 5: Crystals And Meditation For The Third Eye

Crystal Healing is a whole subject in itself but in the context of this book we'll look at specific healing techniques which are recommended for opening the Third Eye and increasing your psychic abilities, along with your spiritual awareness. There are several books available on the subject of crystal healing in general and these may be useful tools to explore as you develop your abilities. For the time being, using the following techniques will help to open and heal your Third Eye.

Crystal Healing Basics

Different types of crystal vibrate with different frequencies of energy and these energies can also be found in each different Chakra. By using appropriate crystals you can help to strengthen this vibration and therefore activate your Third Eye. Stones that are suitable for the purpose include most gemstone (precious or semi-precious) that are colored purple. Several are mentioned in the previous chapter but Amethyst and Indigo are popular options and are widely available online or from New Age or spiritualist stores. The technique is simple; after cleansing and charging your crystal, you simply mentally focus on the crystal and "place" your intention within the stone and, when this is completed, place it in an appropriate location (or carry it with you). These basic steps are outlined below;

1. Cleansing your crystal; this should be done, ideally, in pure or distilled water with natural sea salt added to it. Leave the crystal submerged in the water overnight, for at least eight hours.

2. Charging your crystal; this is normally achieved by placing the crystal in direct sunlight for several hours. For the best effects place the crystal on a window which receives full sunlight (south facing) throughout the day. Although it's possible to leave the crystal for around five hours, the best results will be achieved by placing the crystal on the window as the sun rises

and leaving it in place until sunset. Again, for the most powerful results, do this during summer, when the highest level of exposure to natural sunlight can be achieved.

3. Program your crystal; in a quiet place where you will not be disturbed, make yourself comfortable and lie back, flat on your back. Use a small pillow, if necessary, and then place the cleansed, charged crystal on your forehead, between, but a little above, your eyes. Close your eyes and relax, focusing on your intention for the crystal. In this case, think about the purpose of the Third Eye. State the purpose you require of the crystal clearly; for example say "I wish to open my Third Eye". Vary the statement as you see fit to include increasing your psychic abilities, your spiritual awareness or your clairvoyant skills. Be clear in your intention for the crystal and also keep the statement simple. Repeat the statement several times, keeping this up for a few minutes as a minimum is ideal and the longer the better!

<u>4.</u> Place your crystal appropriately; this is up to you, but many people will keep the crystal under their pillow, or close by in their bedroom. It's also common to carry the programmed crystal with you. This can be done in a pocket or a specially made bag. Neither method is preferable – choose which you feel comfortable with.

Importantly, try to avoid crystals programmed for different purposes from touching each other, to avoid damaging the energy they emit.

Meditation and The Third Eye

Meditation is an ancient practice and forms an essential part of all major – and plenty of minor – spiritual practices. Prayer, reflexion and meditation can be found in as diverse a set of religions as it's possible to imagine. From Jain traditions (one of the oldest still practiced traditions in the world) to "younger" belief systems including Christianity and Islam. Wherever you look, meditation forms an aspect of both worship and spiritual discovery. It should be no surprise then, that it plays an important role in developing, opening and using your Third Eye! In this section we'll take a look at a simple meditation technique that will help you to develop your own Third Eye. For those that are unfamiliar with meditation techniques, we've structured the process in three steps, each building on the other and all working towards opening your Third Eye. Practice each section until you are proficient and then move on to add the next step.

Basic Meditation – Step 1 – Learning to Meditate

1. Create a quiet space to meditate, ensure you will not be disturbed by any intrusions, including excess noise and light. Wear comfortable clothing and ensure that the temperature in the room you are using is also comfortable, neither excessively warm nor cold.

2. Once you are settled comfortably (you can lie or sit, whichever is easier) begin breathing in a slow, deep and rhythmical way. To be sure that you are breathing in deeply enough, breathe through your stomach (pushing it out as you breathe in

and contracting it as you breathe out). Count to four as you breathe in, hold your breath for two and count to four as you breathe out. Breathe in through your nose and out through your mouth.

<u>3.</u>　If you feel tension in any part of your body direct your breathing to that part; imagine the tension dispersing as you breathe out and feel each muscle relax. If you experience thoughts intruding on your meditation simply acknowledge them but don't dwell on them. Allow them to drift through your consciousness but don't stop to focus on any of them.

Basic Meditation - Step 2 - Locating the Third Eye

<u>1.</u>　Once you have mastered basic meditation, described above, you can add the following stages to the process to begin to become aware of your Third Eye. Once you are in a meditative state begin to shift your focus from your breathing to your forehead; think of the feel of it, any wrinkles and the eye brows. Gradually focus on the point above the eyes and to the center of the forehead.

2. Now focus your breathing on this area; imagine energy being drawn into it as you breathe in and any negative energy being dispersed as you breathe out. Gradually you will feel a light tingling sensation in the area of the Third Eye, which indicates that it's awakening and that you have successfully located it.

Basic Meditation – Step 3 – Using a Mantra

Once you can regularly feel the presence of your Third Eye you can add a Mantra to your meditation. Specific mantras in the form of single sounds are associated with each of the Chakras; in this case the sound is "THOH". The word is pronounced as in "though" with the focus on the "th" sound. Tip: you can check online for audio clips of this Mantra to ensure you are pronouncing it correctly. Pronounce the word as you breathe out and try to extend it for as long as possible, take a pause, breathe in and then repeat as you breathe in. Repeat this for several minutes, or longer, and repeat the meditation every day for three to five days. You should begin to feel a clear tingling in the region of your Third Eye – and may initially experience this as a headache. This will pass and after a few days the sensation should feel pleasant and filled with energy.

After repeating the meditation with the Mantra until you can feel this sense of energy in the Third Eye, continue to meditate daily without using the Mantra. Simply breathe energy in to the Third Eye during meditations and expel any negative sensations. Gradually you will find that you experience very vivid dreams, flashes of prediction or psychic moments on a regular basis, along with a deepened sense of intuition and a general rise in creative feelings or expression. At this point you can relax; you've successfully opened your Third Eye!

Chapter 6: Reiki And Your Chakra

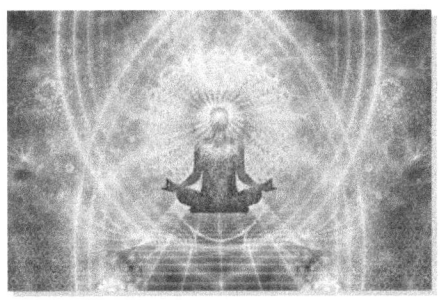

Everywhere around us, there is an energy that is constantly changing. Our bodies soak up this energy like a sponge and it is absorbed through your chakras.

Awareness to the chakras in the human body has been around since before the new age and they play a vital role in yoga.

In Sanskrit, the word chakra literally means "wheel of light" and that is how chakras should be looked at as a gift, especially to those that can see them. When someone can see them, they appear as spinning colored light wheels. Each chakra appears as a different color on the rainbow spectrum.

Each chakra is aligned along the spinal column and they form the backbone that connects the body, mind, and spirit. This network includes several smaller energy centers throughout the body and typically corresponds with acupuncture points.

During a Reiki session, the hands will be placed on the major chakras as well as the secondary chakras, which are typically dysfunctional and discolored or even closed off completely because of problems with one's mind, spirit, or body. It is important to keep these gateways open because if there is a disruption in the energy flow, then one may lead to illness.

When Usui developed his version of Reiki, the Japanese culture did not think of the body's energy in terms of chakras. Instead, they were focused more on the hara which is between the pubic bone and the navel. This area will be the center of the body's gravity. There is also a tanden which is in the center of the chest and just above the brow.

But, the understanding of chakras in ancient times added value to Reiki that was practiced around the world. Today, Reiki is practiced everywhere and it takes into account the importance of chakras.

Reiki treatments are supposed to help clear out energy blockages in the chakras while restoring the flow of one's life force energy. Energy flows in and out of one's aura through the chakras. This aura is a light that envelopes every person. The aura is composed of seven layers, each one dealing with the various aspects of our being. The major chakras create a cone around the core of the spine throughout every layer of our aura.

In one's physical body, each major chakra corresponds with an endocrine gland that helps to control the hormonal balance and a major nerve plexus.

At the base of the spine, there is the root chakra; between the genitals and naval is the sacral chakra; above that is the solar plexus chakra; in the middle of the chest is the heart chakra; in the middle of the neck is the throat chakra; below the brow is the third eye chakra; and at the top of the head is the crown chakra.

There are over a hundred minor chakras in the body as well that play into Reiki.

Balancing Chakras

When your chakras are balanced, you will feel more at peace. You may notice that your chakras are out of balance when you begin to feel ill. Here are some techniques you can use to balance your chakra with Reiki.

Place one hand on the crown chakra and the other on the root chakra.

Move each hand closer and further from the body sensing the chakra energy.

If you feel less energy on one of the chakras, then you can use both hands on that chakra using Reiki to bring the chakra back in its original position.

Keep using Reiki until you feel the same with both hands. You should feel a sense of balance so you know that it is fine to move to the next chakra.

The next session will start with your hand over your third eye chakra and your sacral chakra.

You will repeat the same experience until the chakras are balanced.

Continue moving down the chakras until you have finished balancing all the chakras.

Chapter 7: How To Become A Reiki Channel

The Reikian Future

As stated in chapter 1, we can all be a Reiki channel. There is no age limit, and no condition is required. Reiki is available to everyone, including children, the elderly, and the sick. All of us, in certain moments of our life, go through difficult situations of suffering, both personal and foreign, not only physical or material but also emotional, psychic, and, sometimes, spiritual suffering. We wanted to eliminate the suffering; we would have liked, at least, to be able to minimize that pain or help provide relief to those who were close, and we felt completely helpless. How many times have we thought that if we could have something to interact with and help alleviate suffering, life could be much better. Then, somehow, it comes to our knowledge that Reiki is available to us and that it is inexhaustible.

In that happy moment, it is necessary to look for a qualified Reiki master in one or several systems (Usui, Tibetan, Osho, or Kahuna) and participate in a tuning seminar. Reiki is an energy of love that passes through our hearts and through our heart chakra. When we become a Reiki Channel, we are only a means through which the energy of universal love flows. We realize, after the energy activation promoted by a qualified teacher, that we are able to help and provide help to the neighbor who needs it, being able to flow through our hands the vital, healing, cosmic, spontaneous, and unlimited energy with a simple gesture. It is so simple that we resist believing it. It's incredible!

At that moment, a totally new, different world opens up for us, which, in the beginning, we cannot accept that it could exist. In the meantime, we need to remain alert so as not to allow that recognition to alter our ego, which would hinder our own evolutionary process.

From the moment of initiation, a door is opened within the person that, once passed, introduces it into a new reality. The initiate becomes a true Reiki Energy channel; that is, he will always have contact with that universal energy, and you can apply it whenever you want. And just by laying hands, energy will flow.

The Initiation Process

This process of initiation becomes necessary because, originally, the man kept his energy channels intact, generating happiness and harmony. With the process of forgetting our origin, in the face of extreme individualization and the evolution of feelings of selfishness and pride, we narrow these communication channels, stop using them, and end up not receiving all the energy necessary for our good to live. We come to retain only the energy essential to the sustenance of our biochemical process for survival.

The initiation is a sacred ceremony, and contact is re-established through the teacher who enables it as an energy channel. A true Reiki master receives a series of energy transmissions and is able to activate, apply, and teach others. The Reiki teacher does not exert power over his students. It is simply someone who chose to accept the great responsibility of transmitting to the interested parties the knowledge they acquired in their destiny.

Mikao Usui rediscovered the way to re-religionize the vital energy of the universe. "Religare," that process that was first given the name of initiation, is today called the process of tuning or tuning, indicating that the person is adjusted or tuned to Reiki, similar to the tuning that takes place in a radio or TV, at a certain frequency or station. We can also call this process harmonization because it is a powerful vehicle for the reconciliation of all our bodies.

In the process of initiation, all the channels of force of the body, responsible for the collection and distribution of our energy, are reactivated to function within the original molds, providing the power to heal and harmonize, not only to ourselves but also to all of us who play. Once the initiation is completed, this energy channel will remain open throughout life, preventing the participation and wear of personal energies in the treatments. With initiation, the hands radiate vibrations that flow from the head, when they come into contact with areas in disharmony. The hands are able to cure acute and chronic diseases. This process is complemented by the use of mantras (sounds) and yantras (forms) that have the power to boost energy and break the limitations of time and space.

The initiation is an activation of the higher energy centers (chakras), causing our vibration and frequency to increase and transform, moving to higher levels. That process includes the level of consciousness, and inevitably produces a great transformation that drives our center to climb from the solar plexus to the heart chakra.

The tuning of Level I focuses mainly on the opening of the physical body to be receptive to a large amount of vital energy it will receive. The four tunings that the teacher performs in Level I raise the vibrational frequency of the four centers of the upper part of the human body, which are also known as chakras. The first initiation harmonizes the heart and the thymus gland while tuning the heart chakra with the etheric body.

The second harmonization affects the thyroid gland and, in the etheric field, helps open the throat chakra, which is our communication center. The third initiation affects the so-called third eye, which corresponds to the pituitary gland, our center of high intuition and consciousness, and the hypothalamus, which acts in the control and temperature of the body.

The fourth harmonization increases the opening of the coronary chakra, our communication with the spiritual consciousness, which corresponds to the pineal gland. That final synchronization completes the process, sealing the open channel so that it can remain open for the rest of life, even if we do not use it for a long period of time. Meanwhile, at the moment we decide to use it, it will be at our disposal. During the initiation process, the person being activated may experience a series of sensations, such as: feeling a lot of peace and harmony, a pleasant warmth, a deep relaxation, warmth in the hands, deep sadness, crying, or love. The person can also visualize teachers, see lights, see colors such as blue, violet, gold, and even project into the past. We already had the opportunity to assist many people who visualized disembodied relatives.

The Twenty-One Days of Energy Cleaning

After initiation, it may seem that our condition has worsened or is more serious. Actually, we will be going through a cleaning process that cannot be avoided. This process can lead to serious crises, as old energy blocks will be eradicated. Toxins and impurities considered as energy waste are stored in the human being throughout his life, minimizing the quality of life, and during this elimination, all toxins, and impurities of our physical, mental, emotional, and spiritual bodies will be discarded.

"Cleansing" will occur through feces, urine, sweat, thoughts, dreams, and in the form of negative feelings that were generated. After the removal of these sediments, the body will be able to function more harmoniously and positively.

The Reiki practitioner, after each initiation at different levels of the practice, may feel emotional (anger / love), magnetic (rejection / attraction), mental (thoughts / confusions) and spiritual (construction / destruction) reactions. This process will last a maximum of twenty-one days.

Cleaning, on its way from the coronary center to the heart center, takes about three days. That of the lower centers takes more time, approximately the remaining eighteen days, because they are denser and less rapid vortices.

During this elimination period, it is essential that the self-application be carried out daily to facilitate the cleaning process, mainly positions 1 and 4 of the head, 1 and 3 from the forehead, and 3 and 4 from the back.

During those three weeks, it is advisable to avoid, or at least minimize, the consumption of alcoholic beverages, red meat, and canned goods. Try to eat plenty of water, fruits, legumes, vegetables, and foods high in fiber.

Reiki Systems

The objective of this work is the dissemination, mainly, of the Traditional Reiki System Mikao Usui, or Usui Shiki Ryoho. There are other systems or methods of Reiki or use of the same energy: we can highlight the Osho Reiki, Tibetan System, and the Kahuna Reiki, which we will also talk about later.

Reiki Schools

Before the death of teacher Hawayo Takata, she created a Reiki association that was called AIRA (American International Reiki Association). As a result of divergences in AIRA, in 1982, new associations emerged. Some teachers remained in the AIRA and named Barbara Weber Ray as their great teacher. Others, when they separated, created the "Reiki Alliance," and as Takata had asked, they named Phyllis Lei Furumoto (their granddaughter) as their great teacher.

A third group decided not to accept the orientations and guidelines of the two associations created and decided to take their own path in the interpretation of the technique, and they called themselves traditional or independent teachers, thus forming the "Unlimited Reiki." And still, others formed centers or work centers with identification with the teachers initiated or activated by them.

The responsibility for disseminating Reiki is equally exercised by all teachers, regardless of their relationship with these two main schools. The difference between the two schools is basically that the AIRA divides Reiki into seven grades or levels, calls it "Radiance Technique," and does not accept alterations in its established principles since then, in addition to the fact that its teachers need authorization from the great teacher, currently Dr. Barbara Weber Ray, to start new teachers. The "Reiki Alliance" presents Reiki on three levels, following the line of Dr.

Mikao Usui, the third level can be divided into two sub-levels, as presented in this book. Reiki Alliance teachers recognize other teachers trained by other systems, and their teachers can start other teachers without the permission of the great teacher, currently Phyllis Lei Furumoto (1998).

Both lines are valid and convey the true Reiki; both great teachers were activated by the same teacher, Hawayo Takata, and, as for technique, there is no difference in the transmission itself. Recently, excellent groups and diffusion nuclei of Reiki emerged, which have international projection. We quote below the address of those main schools:

IThe Reiki Alliance
PO BOX 41, 83.810, 140.141
Cataldo, Idaho, USA.

II)American International Reiki Association INC
PO BOX 86038, 33.738
St. Petersburg, Florida, USA.

III)The International Center For Reiki Training 29209

Northwestern HWY, No. 592 Southfield, Michigan, USA.

IV)ASW. und Energiearbeit Zentrum
63329, E. Kastner Str. 72
Egelsbach, Germany

Chapter 8: The Benefits Of Reiki Healing

As one of the oldest healing principles being used today, Reiki is also a natural non-invasive system. This healing method uses the flow of energy that balances mind and body. The benefits are felt by not only patients but the healing professionals as well. Reiki is proven to heal emotional and physical issues, resulting in stress reduction for both patient and practitioner. Reiki techniques are used to heal body and mind, as well as the spirit. It has been a proven tool to help those who are suffering major and minor health problems.

Reiki is often used in hospitals as a complementary therapy for patients that are assisted during outpatient care. Reiki is for everyone, including pets. One of the best benefits of Reiki healing is the reduction of stress. It starts in the immune system which then aids in relaxation to provide better sleep, which wraps back around and helps to improve overall health.

Reiki also helps to create harmony and inner peace. It is also very valuable for those searching for spiritual growth. Reiki also promotes a balance of mind and emotions. With enough treatments, people are able to cope with stress and live a calmer and more peaceful life. This balance also increases mental awareness and memory sharpness. Reiki can heal emotional issues and help to eliminate more severe problems. Reiki helps lessen fear, anger, mood swings, anxiety, and fear. It will also work to heal and strengthen relationships.

Reiki is also known to speed up recovery time from surgery by adding an abundance of energy to the patient and ensuring the body is adjusting to medicines used in treatment. It also aids in the reduction of side-effects. It is also known to relieve migraine pain, arthritis and helps with symptoms of fatigue, insomnia, and asthma. Reiki can also improve and maintain both mental and physical balance.

People are constantly on the go. Time moves quickly, and pressures are constant. We feel the need to speed up, in order to fulfill our obligations or to complete jobs on time, which adds to the stress and pressure on our minds. Our bodies, minds, and spirits are moving into high gear. Life demands this and so does everything around us including family, work, bills, and transportation. Our brains run out of energy fuel, and our bodies suffer. It's really important to stop, re-focus within and let your body, mind, and spirit breathe, so you can concentrate on finding your center and calming down.

Working long hours, dealing with emotional issues, and coping with stress are all examples of where Reiki healing can help because of its positive effects. No matter what your issues in life are, Reiki can be the answer to a better, healthier life and happiness.

Reiki is also working alongside modern medicine. It is used in conjunction with other treatments such as medications and chemotherapy, and helps to reduce and relieve the side effects of other drugs that may be required. It makes for an ideal treatment plan for the reduction of chemotherapy side effects. Reiki can treat emotional disturbances as well including conditions like mood disturbing bipolar disorders.

There are still some conflicting research and findings concerning studies that reported this treatment is known to reduce stress, pain, and anxiety, thereby improving symptoms of depression and fatigue. Reiki principles are showing an increase when it comes to being applied as part of a complete overall physical and emotional care of patients for disease treatments, including more conventional care in U.S. hospitals, as well as holistic healthcare centers.

As yoga and meditation have increased in popularity in the U.S., so has the interest in the Indian Science of Life. This science is over 5,000 years old and is known as "Ayurveda," It has to do with using food, herbs, supplements and a healthy lifestyle to promote an increased lifespan. The theory of Ayurveda is that it can help to heal imbalances in energy types in the body that include the principles known as "***Doshas***" which are comprised of the elements of fire, water, air, ether, and earth.

Many things can disturb the balance of energy such as a diet that is unhealthy, stress, relationships, and even the weather. This imbalance often manifests itself as some type of disease.

Ayurveda is just starting to be studied in the western part of the world. Research has mainly been looking at the Ayurvedic program's effectiveness in treating diseases like anxiety, depression, high blood pressure, and Alzheimer's disease as well as other medical issues. This medicine's use should be supervised by a trained holistic practitioner as some could be harmful, especially if improperly used.

Reflexology is when pressure is applied to particular parts of the body, i.e., hands, ears, and feet, to improve health. This system is called, "body mapping." It is a system that connects pressure points to systems and organs in the human body. Some of the studies discovered that reflexology could be helpful to reduce anxiety, pain, and depression as well as to assist in stress relief and relaxation. Claims have been reported stating that reflexology can treat illnesses such as diabetes and arthritis but they have yet to be verified.

Chapter 9: Chakras And The Aura

THE CHAKRAS

In Sanskrit the word chakra means a spinning wheel. It is possible that the great Indian healers of yesteryears saw the chakras spinning like wheels inside the human body and named them accordingly. Chakras are also known as Spirit Energy Centers. The human body consists of seven major chakras and each chakra has a definite color of its own. Each chakra is also placed in a specific area of the human body, across the human spine starting from the bottom to the top. They are placed thus to monitor the good functioning of the area where they are found.

THE ROOT CHAKRA

The first one is the Root Chakra which is situated at the end of the tail bone exactly between the sex and the anus and its color is red. The Root Chakra controls the body's excretory system that eliminates excess and unnecessary materials from the body fluids in order to maintain health and prevent damage to the body. The dysfunctioning of the Root Chakra will certainly lead to various physical ailments and affliction in that particular area such as constipation, bowel problems, piles, urinary problems, colorectal cancer to name a few. But the Root Chakra has the power to go beyond the area where it is situated in the body. It is a major chakra which controls the human system at all levels, be it physical, emotional, mental, psychic or spiritual. The question you may ask is how can the Root Chakra, placed so low down in the body, have power over and affect man's mental condition? We know that whatever is related to the mind is related to the head and whatever is related to human emotion is related to the heart. Generally all emotional problems tend to be related to the Heart Chakra instead of the Root Chakra. And yet, even as the Root Chakra sits so low in the body, it is one of the most important chakras of the body.

We had earlier spoken about Energy, of Light. The New Science today also accepts the fact that the Universe, including all of its living beings, is made of Energy, not matter. This theory is not new under the sun. Thousands of years ago the ancient Rishis of India proclaimed this theory saying that the Universe is made up of Energy—pure Energy—even before man and Earth came into being. This theory was later taken up by the great Socrates in Europe who said that Energy or Soul is separate from matter.

The 17th Century Newtonian physics which gradually became the corner-stone of science tried to prove later that there is only matter and nothing else. According to Newton, the whole Universe is made of matter and so are we. However the Reiki System of Healing is not stuck in the Newtonian concept. Reiki promotes the ancient theory of the great sages saying that as you probe deeper and deeper into the workings of the billion and billion of atoms of which the human body is made of, you find that the atoms are devoid of matter. There is nothing there—just energy waves.

Had humans realized that they are essentially made up of the two most supreme elements—Light and Energy—they wouldn't most probably want to live in their weighty material world, carrying along a heavy mass of flesh and bones. They would perhaps have opted to be in their Energy form and in the Energy world. But the Creator of all living forms made sure that they loved their outward appearances and their surroundings. And this is the reason why the Chakras are there to control the human body at all levels.

As I was saying earlier, the Root Chakra, the most important one, is there to keep us anchored in our material world. This is also the reason why we say that the Root Chakra is the base of our body because it connects us to our material selves and attracts us to live in our physical body. If ever the Root Chakra becomes weak or stops spinning or the person gets disconnected with his Root Chakra, then that person is bound to get disconnected with the material world. Such people are generally found to either commit suicide or phase away slowly with no desire to live further. With Reiki it is possible to heal such people by activating the Root Chakra. When healing occurs and this Chakra is restored, the patient starts feeling better in his material body and rediscovers the taste of being alive. Thus it is unquestionable that the Root Chakra affects us at both the physical and mental levels.

The same can be said for all the other chakras of the body.

THE SACRAL CHAKRA

The second chakra is the Sacral Chakra which is of orange color. The Sacral Chakra, which is also known as the creativity and the sexual chakra, sees to the good functioning of all our reproductive organs. We daily encounter cases— sometimes severe—of female infertility where able-bodied women, with healthy reproductive organs, cannot still reproduce and have babies and that in spite of medical treatments. Infertility can also affect men, for both men and women can be infertile.

Reiki can definitely heal such patients. Practice of Reiki activates the weak Sacral Chakra and eventually the related organs which in most cases have been dormant and non-functional. With Reiki Healing System, the Sacral Chakra is restored to spinning at its full original capacity and facilitates the process of pregnancy and the production of offspring.

THE SOLAR PLEXUS CHAKRA

The third chakra is the Solar Plexus Chakra, which is of yellow color is located between the human navel and the solar plexus, is known as our power storehouse. It is considered to be the core of our identity, our personality and our ego. The Solar Plexus Chakra is also connected with our digestive system in its entirety, anchoring all the upper and lower chakras.

THE HEART CHAKRA

The fourth is the green Heart Chakra which physically controls the arterial system that carries blood from the heart to the organs. According to Reiki, the Heart Chakra controls everything related to our emotions.

THE THROAT CHAKRA

The fifth is the Throat Chakra which has the blue color and is located in the region of the neck. This Chakra physically governs the anatomical regions of the thyroid, parathyroid, mouth, larynx, jaw, mouth, tongue and neck. Known as the first of the three spiritual chakras, the Throat Chakra is also connected with our behavioral patterns and our communications with others. There are people who simply cannot communicate easily; not that they are dumb-headed or dim-witted, but they still display difficulties while communicating freely. Such people are believed to have problems with their Throat Chakra. Once this Chakra is healed and restored, the person regains their capacity to speak, listen and express themselves from a higher form of communication.

THE Brow CHAKRA

The Brow Chakra is the sixth chakra of the human body and is located in the forehead between the eyes. It is often referred to as the Third Eye and it governs the human eyes both at the physical and the spiritual levels. The Brow Chakra is also most active on other levels like intuition, psychic ability, intelligence and memory among others.

THE CROWN CHAKRA

The last and one of the most important chakras of the human body is the Crown Chakra. It is placed exactly on the top of the head on the crown. The Crown Chakra is slightly different from the rest of the chakras because it is an open chakra. This chakra is believed to be just like a funnel, not too long, located on the head, which draws in Life-force Energy at all times and throughout life from the Universe to feed and reinforce the other chakras of the body. Just like the mouth needs food to keep the physical body alive, The Crown Chakra also needs Life-force Energy to constantly feed the other chakras and keep them in good working condition.

We all know that a baby is born with two soft spots, known as fontanelles (head bones) on its head. Eventually, as the baby grows these head bones meet and fuse and the soft spots close. Reiki practitioners claim that these fontanelles in an infant remain connected with its Energy world for quite a few months after its birth. Babies, it is believed, can see things that grownups cannot. However as they grow up, the infants lose their extra-sight abilities. Scientists have been trying to research baby behavior in this field. Even animals are said to behold things that adults cannot see. It is also believed that animals, unlike human beings who possess five senses, have further perceptive abilities that enable them to experience the world in ways we can hardly imagine. Animals, young or old, are believed to be gifted with a sixth sense that human beings either don't have or they have lost it through disregard and long neglect.

The human baby, as it grows up starts thinking about right and wrong and begins to experience emotions such as jealousy, anger, revenge—all negative energies—which accumulate in its Brow Chakra as he grows up. So, generally, the Life-force Energy which flows down through the human Crown Chakra into the body to nourish the other chakras is mostly used to cleanse the Brow Chakra of all its impurities and it negative energies before it can move further on.

Therefore, it is good to remember that the Universal Energy, of which we are made, is divine and positive. However, when negative energy accumulates excessively in the Brow Chakra, it becomes difficult to cleanse it the funnel-like opening on top of the crown, starts to shrink, with little or no energy passing through it. Obviously when there is no incoming Energy from the Crown Chakra, the lower chakras of the body progressively become weak, shrink and become non-functional. The result—the body becomes affected with a lot of known and unknown predicaments. This is the reason why we should keep the Brow Chakra, which is in fact our mind and our ego, clear of all negative thoughts. This is where prayers come in. We are taught to pray from a tender age. Prayer can bring lasting peace and positive change in our lives. While praying we always look up to the Almighty, to the skies while praying. This is because we all know the source from which we have emanated. The Life-giving Energy comes from the Universe, not from the material world. We are also taught to search for God within us. The essence of it all is that the Energy which feeds us with life is indeed the god for us, whatever name we give Him.

There is one more important function that the Crown Chakra fulfills and that is keeping the two hemispheres of the brain in perfect balance. People with weakened Crown Chakra show common signs of bipolar problems like epilepsy, or schizophrenia and so forth.

THE AURA

Since most ancient times there have been illustrations, paintings, sculptures of different spiritual leaders across various cultures and traditions of the world. Each is special, different in its own way.

However, the one thing common among all of them is halo of light that surrounds their heads. This brilliant halo is known as the Aura—the Energy Field.

Reiki practitioners define Aura in more comprehensible terms. According to them, all chakras, while spinning, radiate a color––their own respective colors--—as they go about their work in the body. The Root Chakra radiates red color; the Sacral Chakra will beam orange color and so on. Thus, all the chakras, each gleaming and glowing in its own color, form a rainbow-like bright Energy sparkling from the wheel in the body and extending to the outer body creating a kind of colorful energy-shield round our body. This rainbow-like bright emanation surrounding the body of a living creature is called the Aura. The Aura, according to Reiki practitioners, is the very Essence of the individual. The Aura can be discerned by people with special sensibilities.

The Aura, radiating from within, can extend to several inches or even several feet in some cases outside the shell of the body. The Picture above depicts the human body surrounded by a rainbow-like energy—the Aura. It is as if the body is encased in a luminous egg-shell. However, the Aura cannot be generally beheld through the naked eye. How then, can one prove that the aura exists?

For quite a long time Science rejected the concept of the Aura. However, today, with the development of Hi-tech electronic gadgets and instruments, it has become possible to detect and capture a glimpse of the human aura. Research on capturing this subtle energy field through electronic instruments was started in the 1960s by a professor called Semyon Kirlian, a Czech scientist and researcher, who, while wanting to ameliorate the performance of the X-ray machine, accidentally discovered that if an object on a photographic plate is linked to a basis of high voltage, small radiance (created by the powerful electric field at the edges of the object) generate a reflection on the photographic plate.

Although Dr Kirlian is given credit for being the first researcher to invent a technical device which show the human aura, we have proof that long before him another device, known as the Kilner Goggles had already been invented by a renowned British physician named Walter John Kilner (1847-1920). He was also a member of the Royal College of Physicians. He did a lot of research on the human Aura which he called 'the Etheric Double'. He even published his first book on the subject entitled 'The Human Atmosphere', which was revised and republished as 'The Human Aura' after his death in 192o.

Kilner Goggles and Kirlian's Verographs are pretty much in use even today. But we all have (if we apply ourselves) the potential to perceive the Aura without the help of any device. Reiki Channels can do it easily, for they are Light Workers. Of course to be able to detect the aura one needs time, special exercises and hard work before the final goal is achieved. Perceiving or feeling the Aura of a patient without any device is a great advantage for a Reiki Healer.

Animal Aura

As far as the animal aura is concerned, according to Reiki, animals also remain open to the Universal Life-force Energy throughout their life. One may ask why then do animals get sick and die early? Some animals even suffer a lot before dying. One possible answer may be that animals get sick probably because of their close interactions and connections with human beings. We now know that all human beings do not have clean, strong and healthy auras. Some people are themselves very sick when they acquire pets. Living in their proximity, the pets progressively absorb their master's unhealthy energy and ultimately fall sick. Animals living in their natural habitat, far away from humans and left on their own do not face health problems and they live long lives.

Chapter 10: Using Reiki With Others

After working with yourself for a while, you will find that Reiki comes incredibly natural to you. Once you have reached the stage where you feel completely confident in this practice, you will be able to start using Reiki with others. The major benefit is that the life force will be felt in the giver and the receiver during practice. You can help your family and friends, while simultaneously reaping the benefits of Reiki yourself.

Why You Should Practice with Others

The relationship formed between two entities practicing Reiki is often referred to as a healing alliance. The most common experience of the giver is harmony. As you form alliances with others, you will find more peace and harmony in your own life. You may also experience feelings of oneness with others or nature or the world as a whole.

What To Do

You will find that there are a number of similarities between the way you would practice Reiki on yourself and the way that you would practice it on someone else.

Step #1: Discovering Their Intent

In order for Reiki practice to be effective for the other person, you must be very clear about what they are expecting from the session. The best way to do this is to have a long conversation beforehand about the other person's intentions. Ask questions like:

How would you like to benefit from Reiki treatment?

Do you have any specific ailments or illnesses?

What if Reiki brings a sense of positivity to your life?

Do you have a sense of purpose in life?

Are there any pressing issues on your mind?

How is your life at home? At work?

Do you feel stressed?

Asking open-ended questions like these gives you and the receiver the chance to explore their deepest desires without much restriction. As you uncover what they desire most, ask follow-up questions until you have a clear picture of their intent before you begin Reiki practice. In order to establish a sense of trust, it is important to make it clear that you will not repeat anything said in a Reiki session to anyone else. This may make your partner more comfortable.

Step #2: Active Practice

In the initial phases of the Reiki session, you will practice in the same way that you would with yourself. You will either place your hands on the six hands positioned found in the previous chapter or place your hands on each of the seven chakras.

Once you have finished this, you will do something known as spiraling. Take your left hand and place it on the right shoulder. Take your right hand and point your middle and index finger outward. Use these to draw counterclockwise spirals, starting at the left shoulder and moving toward the tip of the left hand. Then, start at the shoulder again and move toward the left foot. You will repeat this on the right side. This is intended to balance the energy before flipping the patient to heal the back chakras.

Once you have asked your healing partner to turn so they are laying on their stomach, hold your hands above the body and perform a Byosen scan again, paying close attention to the chakras located above the back brow and the lower back. Now, stand with your hands about six inches above either of these chakras. Feel the flow of energy between each until they feel balanced.

Next, take the middle and index fingers of your right hand and make a "V" shape. Keeping your hand on the left shoulder, draw a line that spans between the throat and root chakras. Pause for a moment at the back chakra and repeat this process twice more. Then, awaken your partner.

Step #3: How to Know if It is Working

Sometimes, you will not receive confirmation that the Reiki session is doing what it is intended to do until a day or even a week after the session. This is especially true of earlier practices, which will not be as strong in nature. In other cases, you will feel sensations through the course of the situation, which may include tingling, vibration, or temperature changes. Sometimes the sensations of Reiki will be felt together and other times the giver and receiver will experience this as opposites, such as one feeling hot and the other feeling cold. Whether you do or do not experience something, do not lose faith that the Reiki session is working. It will work, but sometimes the results take time.

A Few Tips to Keep in Mind When Practicing Reiki with Others

#1: It Is Never Okay to Make Promises

There are a number of factors that affect how effective a Reiki practice is for the people involved. As the giver, you must not make promises for how the session will end. You cannot guarantee that the receiver will find confidence or be healed in some way. All that you can do is help them set the intent for the session and then provide the practice in the best way you can. Other than that, the results are going to be up to them.

#2: Start with Willing Friends and Family Members

The receiver does not have to be sick or anxious in order to reap benefits from a Reiki session. This means that you can practice with anyone, as long as they have an open mind. Remind your willing participant that their results are going to rely heavily on their state of mind and intent during practice. Finally, be sure that they know that the results are always unique to the person and their situation, so you cannot guarantee anything.

#3: Practice with Plants and Animals

The spiritual life force of Reiki flows through every living being, including plants and animals. If the person that you practice with is unavailable, try with a pet or even a plant. While the technique will not be exactly the same, try to use the same visualization of the chakras as an internal tube of light. The chakras will align along this tube.

#4: Remember That You Cannot Control the Entire Session

As the healer in the Reiki practice, you do not have much control over the results. Imagine for a moment that you are a boat taking spices to India. If the sailors hit something and the boat drowns, is it the fault of the boat? No, it is not. In this situation, you are the boat. You can transport the Reiki energy to the receiver, but you cannot make it improve their life. If they are holding on to past grudges or do not honestly feel that Reiki will work, it is not going to benefit them as much as they would like it to. Additionally, it may take more than one Reiki session for the benefits to be felt as fully as they would like.

Chapter 11: The Seven Chakras

In the practice of Reiki, much like Yoga, chakras come into play and are actually one of the most important aspects of it. In order to understand energy flow and how you can make use of it in your daily life, familiarizing yourself with the seven (7) chakras would be among the first steps.

So what are they?

The seven chakras are basically centers of energy within our bodies. They are aligned with our spine and are also associated with our feelings, as well as behavioral and emotional characteristics. Each of these chakras is associated with an internal organ and its bodily function. Typically, they are represented by a particular color as well as a 1 to 7 numbering system. The more sensual aspects of these energy centers also depend on the doctrine and interpretation of different things such as sounds and shapes - including the human's development from the time of conception to maturity.

What is their importance?

It has been said that if the chakras are clear, a person's physical, spiritual, and mental being are also healthy. On the other hand, if it becomes blocked then all of the related functions as well as emotions are also significantly affected. It might lead to bouts of depression, lethargy, and anxiety caused by an imbalance when other chakras are forced to compensate. You can apply Reiki to the affected chakra points when feeling stressed, weak, ill, or in pain to remedy the situation.

The Seven Chakras with their locations and color representations are:

Root or Base – found at the bottom of the pelvis consisting of several organs (kidneys, adrenal glands, leg bones, large intestines, rectum, and spinal column) and represented by the color RED. This chakra keeps a person grounded to his/her physical existence or SURVIVAL.

Sacrum - found just below the navel area consisting of the whole reproductive system including the bladder and spleen.

This is represented by the color ORANGE and is said to fuel one's creativity, emotions, and SEXUALITY.

Solar Plexus – found in the area between the navel and sternum or the central vertical bone of your ribcage affecting the liver, stomach, gall bladder, small intestines, and pancreas. This is represented by the color YELLOW and is associated with a person's intellectual processes. This is also the seat of POWER which when opened and balanced can transform all your aspirations and hopes into reality.

Heart – found at the center of your chest and controls many of the functions associated with the circulatory system (heart, including the arms, lower lungs, skin, and the thymus gland). This is represented by the color GREEN and creates the link from the physical world towards spiritual existence. It is also the center of our emotions, especially the emotion of LOVE.

Throat – found at the base of your neck and controls the thyroid gland, throat, jaw, upper lungs, and vocal chords. It may also affect the digestive system. This is represented by the color SKY BLUE and governs a person's COMMUNICATION ability. This chakra also inspires mental creativity.

Third Eye – found at the brows between your eyes or the center of the lower forehead and involves the organs in the head and central nervous system (brain, nose, face, eyes, and pituitary gland). This is represented by the color INDIGO BLUE and is believed to open one's INTUITION. This chakra allows a person to visualize and even create visions beyond ordinary sight.

Crown – found at the topmost part of your head and corresponds to the person's whole being as well as our direct connection to the spirit. This chakra is represented by the color VIOLET (or sometimes WHITE) and is believed to lead the way on the path towards universal existence or SPIRITUALITY. This chakra also allows us to experience inner peace and opens the path towards spiritual wisdom including the enhancement of one's psychic abilities.

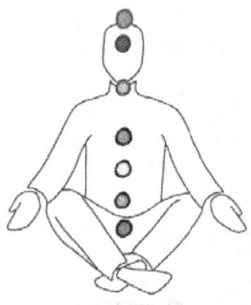

To summarize, the lower chakras are the ones that govern our most basic instincts, relating to both survival as well as our very physical self. The higher chakras are the ones that govern our feelings and mental characteristics, which are both related to our consciousness and thought. The central chakra, the heart, works as a bridge between the two and is associated with physical as well as emotional feelings. The seven chakras play a very crucial role in Reiki and in almost all of the traditional healing arts. Our ailments or illnesses are essentially caused by an imbalance or deficiency in any of these chakras. Reiki aims to clear, open, and balance these energy points to achieve health, overall wellness, and peace.

Chapter 12: Forgiveness

There may be times when your or the client neither one feel as if anything has taken place. This is because the power of Reiki is very dependent on the receiver letting go of past hurts and negative thoughts and feeling. These thoughts and feelings may even be subconscious but they have to be released.

If this happens you need to provide a bit of counseling to your client, direct them toward positive thinking and positive living, refer them to a good councilor if you feel you cannot help them move past the issues and explain to them that these issues are holding them back from receiving the benefits of Reiki.

Often times you can feel it when you lay your hands on a person, sometimes when you enter the room with the person you can feel it if the negativity is strong enough.

One thing I have seen done is that a questionnaire is filled out before each session asking questions like:

Do you harbor any un-forgiveness against anyone for any reason?

Do you feel that you are a mostly positive or mostly negative person?

There were a total of about 10 questions reworded but trying to get the same answer of whether the client was holding onto any negative feelings. If they are you may want to talk to them before the session and explain how the negativity affects the power of Reiki.

You can offer them a free MP3 or even CD discussing positive affirmations and living a positive life and explain that this is just part of the process.

You can also explain to them that they can go ahead and go through a Reiki session and the energy may help work out these deep issues or negative thoughts they are holding onto. While Reiki works on the deeper issues, they may see a reduction in the symptoms they are having to deal with but this can cause the process to take longer than it would if they worked on forgiveness and positive living.

If you find that what you were once doing does not seem to be working for your clients and that your self Reiki is not as strong as it used to be you may feel that your Reiki energy is diminishing. The fact is that the energy you receive is there for life what has happened is that you have an area of your life that has become unbalanced.

Many people give up Reiki when this happens because they really do not understand what is going on. I want to make sure that if this happens to you that you understand what is happening and do not stop helping others with Reiki, all you have to do is figure out a way to rebalance your life. Sometimes this may mean taking some time away from practicing Reiki on others and focusing only on self Reiki once again or it may mean dealing with a negative situation in your life that you have allowed to go on for too long.

Either way if you feel your Reiki diminishing, understand this is not a punishment or the end for you. It is just unbalance in your life.

I spoke briefly earlier about a practitioner taking on the clients symptoms. This is another reason why people become discouraged and stop practicing. The only time you will take on another persons symptoms is when you allow yourself to. You see nothing happens in our lives unless we allow it to happen. If you have strong feelings for the client or a desire to help them with a specific issue you may find that you are taking on their symptoms just to make them happy. This often happens with those who work with very sick loved ones.

This also happens to those who feel like they have to prove that they really can help their clients. Instead of letting Reiki work through them, they are often trying to force something to happen, when they try to control the Reiki energy it opens them up to taking on the negativity of the client. The only way to deal with this is to never feel like you have to produce results, this is the job of Reiki, remember you are just a vessel for the energy, it is not you who is doing the healing.

There are also symbols that can be used from accent Reiki that are said to prove protection for those who are unable to stop themselves from taking on their clients symptoms. What you would do is draw a power symbol in the palm of each hand before each session.

I tend to steer away from this because people are still very leery when it comes to any type of symbol that may contain power and may be scared away from Reiki thinking it is evil.

You can draw the symbol instead on the core of your body which is said to help protect you as well. You can also use affirmations to help with this. Before each session you will have some form of meditation or a ritual that you do for yourself to help you prepare, all you have to do is add to this. You will repeat out loud that you will not take on the negativity of your client, you choose not to allow that negativity to affect you.

It really is that simple. Reiki is not mysterious and it is not magic if you work to keep yourself positive and balanced you can help those who need it.

Chapter 13: How Can You Experience Magnificence?

So, how can you experience magnificence when magnificence is all there is?

How can you experience beauty, when beauty is all there is?

How can you experience up when up is all there is or down when down is all there is?

It's just not possible.

And you knew this.

You knew that to have the experiences that you desired, it was going to be necessary to change everything.

So that is what you did!

The opposite has to exist

You knew that to have the experience of anything, the opposite of what you are wanting to experience would have to exist too. But at this point there was only you, there was in effect, no not you.

So you decided to do the only thing you could do to accomplish what you desired, you decided to divide yourself.

Not too difficult a task for the only and most powerful force in existence, you'd think.

But wait…

Could dividing into just two parts provide all the experiences you wished to experience?

Sure, it would now be possible for one part of you to look back at the other part, but what would that part see?

Well, one part of magnificence would be able to see the other part of magnificence looking back, which would be good, wouldn't it?

After all that's exactly what you wanted.

Well, yes, but only partly. It would only be possible for one part of magnificence to see the other part of magnificence from the perspective of, err… well… magnificence.

Do you understand this concept?

We hope so, but if it hasn't quite clicked into place try considering it like this.

Imagine yourself as being one half of an apple looking back at the other half of yourself...

You can only see the other part from the perspective, and understanding that you already have - which is what you've gained from being an apple.

Because an apple is all you are.

You are not and never have been, say, an orange. And you cannot, therefore, consider the apple from the understanding - the perspective - of an orange.

Got it?

No? Try this then.

If you were completely brown and you lived in a brown world where everything was absolutely brown.

Yes everything - and the same shade of brown too...

Your clothes, furniture, house, décor, car, the road, grass, trees, sky, sun, sea etc. etc.

Have you got the picture?

There's no other colour in your world except brown. Would you be able to understand, to perceive, what it would be like to live in our own multi-coloured world?

Now please don't say, "Well, that makes it as clear as mud".

If you're still not quite sure, re-read the paragraphs above a few more times, and we know you'll finally get it.

It was necessary to divide

Okay then, so it was necessary to divide and into more than two parts, but these parts had to be – different parts, as well.

Now the fundamental problem with this is...

...how do you get a consciousness, which is one thing to become a consciousness, which is something else?

If you are, say, Mary Smith, how do you become Sarah Jones? Yes it would be possible to emulate an actress and pretend to become Sarah Jones.

But are you then really Sarah Jones?

Not really.

You would just be Mary Smith pretending to be Sarah Jones but still using the general perspectives, the general understandings, of Mary Smith.

Everything that you did would be influenced by that major part of you which was really Mary Smith.

Memory Loss

But hold on a minute, what if you had amnesia?

What if you absolutely, totally and utterly forgot who you were?

Yes, now that would work wouldn't it?

If people lose their memories they can become, not just act like, but actually become, a changed person. Their perspectives, their outlook, on life can become quite different.

Ah-ha, this was a good plan, and it was a plan that might just work.

And so it was decided that a portion of this extraordinarily powerful energy would split itself into an infinite number of particles.

Every particle containing within it the essence of the whole, rather like the pieces of a broken hologram, but carrying no conscious memory of this fact.

(If a picture in holographic form of, say a vase, is shattered, every individual piece of the broken hologram carries within it a complete picture of the whole vase.)

This provided the potential for each individual particle to become totally different, and appear to be totally separate from every other particle as well.

So, now it would be possible to experience your magnificence in the very practical way you desired.

The energetic universe begins

So, in an explosion of incredible magnitude the ONE instantly became the many. The universe, the one-verse, was born. Suddenly there was, for the first time, a here and a there. There was an up and a down, a now and a then, a near and a far...

...everything your heart desired.

Well, perhaps not quite your heart, for that little part of you was yet to come - but you know what we mean.

All these centillions of little particles of consciousness - these little chips off the old block - became us.

They became all there is and all there isn't. All the matter and all the anti-matter.

WOW!

This, as you can see, aligns itself quite nicely with the widely accepted theory that the universe began with the Big Bang.

And for us it answers all the questions on creation it's necessary to ask.

But you are quite welcome to go on questioning, if what we've said doesn't 'sit right' with you.

You might still have your own theories of All That Is and the universe, and we honour those beliefs. If you're still not sure, we would suggest you meditate on it, and remember it your own way.

In other words re-member - put the pieces back together - in a way that fits your own internal pattern.

Because, at the end of the day - for each individual - it really does come down to just one thing...

Belief!

Yes, that's right, just belief or more precisely, BEING LIEF.

You see the word lief means: gladly, willingly, happily, readily. And it's no accident how this word evolved.

It's asking you to BE lief. So gladly, willingly, happily, readily accept the possibility of being All That Is.

Just – Be, just BE - lief.

The thought of creation

So, we, as individuals, originated from a thought, which All That Is had had about who All That Is was.

Because All That Is is always unfolding too! We evolved as a concept during the thought processes of All That Is.

All That Is imagined what it would be like to experience being All That Is.

And in doing so created us!

We were created in God's imagination. In God's IMAGE-ination. And the notion of us being created in God's image was born too, along with us.

Now what did we, as little bright sparks of the creator, have to do in order to experience being All That Is?

Well, as always, the answer was in the question.

We didn't have to DO anything. We wanted to experience BEING All That Is. So we became human BEINGS not human doings.

We became Beings of energy, Beings of light, Beings of thought, Beings of All That Is.

And we created a whole universe of energy, of light, of thought, of sound, of All That Is in which to play whilst experiencing our Being-ness.

The physical universe begins

With the creation of this energetic universe there also came two choices of experience for us.

We could experience a physical or a non-physical reality.

Choosing a physical reality meant slowing down the energy around us until it took on a denser form. A bit like taking steam and slowing it down until it becomes water and then slowing it down some more until it becomes ice.

Many of us made the choice to experience physical realities.

So we slowed the energy until it coalesced into the manifestation of the physical universe we inhabit today.

And we did this through the power of thought.

By the way, every particle in the universe responds to our thoughts, but more of this anon.

Now, as it was necessary for us to interact with this physical reality we also had to create the means for this to happen.

So, we created for ourselves physical bodies.

And these physical bodies we created for our-selves also required the slowing down of our divine energy. You see, the energy of All That Is, of which we are, oscillates, vibrates, at incredible speed.

In order for us to have physical experience, this energy has to be stepped down slower and slower and slower until we achieve a physical density.

Or to be more precise what we perceive to be a physical density.

Our various bodies The slowing of our energy begins at the level of the divine and finishes, for us, at the level of the physical.

In between these levels, like the layers of an onion, are the energy images of several other bodies.

These bodies, or step-down energy images as they can be more accurately called, have been detected by clairvoyants and psychics throughout the ages and have been given many different names.

To better understand these phenomena, think about having seen a wrongly exposed photograph.

It can create a double and sometimes triple image, giving the impression of seeing a body within a body.

Impression, actually, is a very good description of what is occurring.

For at every point of the energy step-down procedure, an impression is left as it interacts with the surrounding energy field.

This is because the universe is going through the very same step-down procedures, thereby creating many other separate realities where we can also have experiences.

Chapter 14: Improve Your Life With Reiki

Reiki is something which you can do every day on your own. You just need the right direction and you will be good to go. Reiki has helped many people with sustaining their life in a good manner. People who have been practicing Reiki tend to love it and they include it as an essential part of their life. The energy of Reiki connects everyone to it and gives a power to keep it going. You will be able to see a huge difference in your life by creating a new level of creativity and innovation around yourself. There are somethings which you can do in order to improve your life with Reiki. If you are someone who is going through a hard time and do not understand what to do with life, this is the time to get Reiki in your life. It will help you to stay focused and you will be able to make the right decisions.

There are times in life where you have to make big decisions and if you do not have the will power to make the small daily decisions easily then you will be a complete mess during the big decisions time. Check out the amazing ways of Reiki through which you can excel and improve your life towards betterment.

23. Wake up with Reiki

When you wake up, the first thing which should be on your mind is Reiki. You need to understand the need of Reiki and make sure to start your day with it. Choose any exercise and practice it every morning. You will see that you will have the best day when you do this in the morning and leave for work or school. Make sure to set your alarm a bit earlier than you wake up normally and make it a part of your routine that without it, you cannot start your day so do not forget Reiki at all.

24. Practice Reiki with food

The food which you eat should be blessed with it. So make sure to start with the reminder of Reiki in your inner self and make sure to energize yourself with it. You will notice that the food you eat, even if it is limited will be beneficial for you and will be enough for you as well. It will improve your energy as well you will feel light on your stomach even if you have eaten a lot.

25. Meditation with Reiki

Meditation allows you to concentrate better and helps you getting better. You get more intelligent and thoughtful through meditation. You need to take out time to meditate with Reiki so that you can stay calm and have a positive impact on the people who are around you. You will surely benefit with Reiki but the people around you will also have your vibes and you will see how effective that will be for you. You will have less conflicts with the people. You will not really care who says what or will be less interested in any kind of complications.

26. Pets love Reiki

If you have a pet then they would love reiki so you can practice it with them also. By keeping your hand on them, they will get the vibes from you and you will see how calm they will be. They will be listening to you and won't be a mess for you. They stay settled at their place by doing what they have to without disturbing you much. It has a healing power for every soul whether it is a pet or a human soul. You can convey the Reiki through giving them food or by placing hand on them or by their toys with which they play around.

27. Traveling

When you are traveling somewhere alone or with the family then consider to make use of the Reiki before getting on the trip. It is better that you know about it and you make a use of it before getting on the road trip especially. Road trips are adventurous as well as dangerous which can stress you out so make sure to get a complete hold of it by making proper cautions.

28. Complete Emotions

It helps you keep the balance on your emotions such as at times you are angry but you do not have to show the anger but have to show that you are smiling. Well, by Reiki you can learn how to react and control the emotions by giving out the complete emotion which is necessary according to the situation. You will be able to think quickly and make the decisions right instant that what you have to do rather than thinking after it that you could have done that.

29. Reiki – Spiritual

The life force will be increased through reiki and you will see that when you go through it actually. Some people do not believe on the words, until they have experienced it themselves so make sure to try it yourself and see how amazing it is spiritually. It will raise your energy, forgiveness and gratitude to another level which you would not have imagined.

30. Reiki – Nature

Spend some time with the nature such as go visit some waterfalls, sit in the lawn, play with the flowers or water your plants. It will create another zone of energy for you and you will get the feeling like no other in the world.

Chapter 15: What To Expect From A Reiki Session

Since reiki started out as a type of folk medicine, there is no actual standard involved—though different schools have come up with their own protocols. Some practitioners will jump into a session, trusting in their instincts and faith in a higher power to guide them. Most, however, prefer to engage in some form of pre-consultation. Still others might ask you to sign a consent form before doing a session. Some charge a fee, while others don't.

Most reiki practitioners set aside a specific place where they work. If they come to your home or to a clinic which allows them to operate, they usually (but not always) bring something to create a sense of sacred space. This can be anything from soothing music to incense, as well as symbols (more on this later, or you can go directly to Chapter 7).

All reiki sessions are done with you fully clothed, either seated or lying down on a table. If the latter, you will usually start out by lying on your back and end up lying face down. It's important to let the practitioner know if you have certain needs, however. If breathing is difficult when lying face down, for example, be sure to tell the practitioner beforehand.

The twelve positions cited in the previous chapter will be the primary focus of a reiki practitioner. Depending on their skill set and instinct, they may move to other parts of your body, as well. A full session can last anywhere from ten minutes to as long as ninety minutes, depending on their assessment.

While some reiki practitioners will touch you, others won't. Still others will touch you at some points and remove their hands from others while holding them palms down. Even when not touching you, they believe they are able to direct the ki to that particular spot. Under no circumstances is kneading or stroking involved, since reiki is not a massage.

You should feel relaxed throughout the session, so it's alright if you fall asleep. You will of course be woken up when you need to turn over. Some claim to feel a tingling at some spots, which is the ki doing its job. Do not expect a diagnosis after your session is over. That is not a practitioner's job, nor are they qualified to give one, unless they're also practicing doctors who include reiki in their treatments. Some may give you practical advice, such as drinking more water or taking it easy. That said, you should be wary if they start recommending various prescriptions or suggest you buy something.

You should feel refreshed after a session, but if you feel tired, it's not a bad thing. Different people react to a session differently, depending on individual conditions and circumstances.

While some feel changes after a single session, four is the traditional recommendation of many schools. These are usually done over four consecutive days, but it will also depend on your availability, as well as that of the practitioner. You do not have to have all four sessions from the same practitioner and should be wary if they insist that you do.

Chapter 16: Reiki Healing And Self-Healing

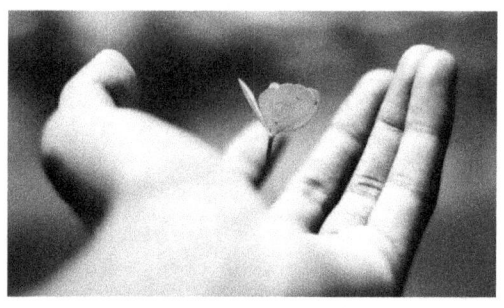

Reiki energy healing is a profoundly powerful tool when healing yourself and also when healing others. It might seem easier to seek out a Reiki practitioner, however, there are different benefits to performing Reiki sessions on yourself.

That being said, there are also benefits to receiving Reiki sessions from practitioners as well. Depending on what your goals are, what your intentions are, and what you have been feeling or going through, is going to be a factor when looking at what method is going to work best for you.

When all said and done, generally utilizing a combination of the ways you can receive and apply Reiki is going to be of the greatest benefit. Of course, the best and most powerful healing comes from within, so implementing daily self-treatment Reiki sessions is always going to be encouraged and recommended.

Depending on where you live, you might find it difficult to find a Reiki practitioner. That isn't necessarily a bad thing. Many Reiki practitioners offer distance and online services and sessions. A distance Reiki session is just as powerful as an in-person session and can yield the same results. Some people find distance sessions to be preferred as they tend to have a little more flexibility around busy or strict schedules.

There are some basic and overall benefits of Reiki healing. The most profound and common benefits that you can receive from Reiki treatments include:

Promoting harmony and balance

Promotes deep relaxation, allowing the body to release stress and tension

Aligns energy imbalances and promotes a balance between body, mind, and spirit

Cleanses the body and organs of toxins and boosts the immune system

Clears the mind and improves focus

Grounds and centers

Assists with sleep

Improves the body's ability to heal itself

Relieves pain and supports healing of the physical body

Guides in spiritual growth and emotional cleansing

Compliments medical treatments and therapies for other conditions

Along with well documented benefits of Reiki energy healing, there are also some disease and conditions that have been known to be benefited when treated with Reiki alongside their medical treatments.

Some common medical diagnoses that have shown improvement or been benefited with Reiki include:

Cancer

Heart Disease

Anxiety

Depression

Chronic Pain
Infertility
Neurodegenerative Diseases
Autism
Crohn's Disease
Fatigue Syndromes

The uses for Reiki healing are innumerable. Even when just seeking to improve your awareness, personal power, and raising your energetic vibration, Reiki becomes such an asset in every day life. There are thousands of reasons to use Reiki energy to heal yourself and very few reasons not to.

The rest of this chapter is going to take a look at different ways Reiki energy can be used for healing, their differences, and their potential benefits. Overtime, you will learn to follow your intuition and the wisdom of Reiki to follow the path that is best for you. Having the correct knowledge and information on different types of Reiki healing sessions is going to help you on that path.

Self- Treatment Sessions

A self-treatment session with Reiki energy can be performed after you receive your Reiki Level I attunement ceremony. In a later chapter, the hand positions for a self-treatment session will be covered, but you can always adapt and change the hand positions to whatever feels right or comfortable.

When performing a Reiki self-treatment, you'll want to make sure that you are in a quiet, relaxed space where you can be undisturbed for around forty-five minutes. This is one benefit to self-treatment sessions, you have more control over how long the session will last. You will also be able to fit them in on your own schedule rather than trying to coordinate with a practitioner and their schedule.

While you can be sitting up or lying down for a Reiki self-treatment, if you are prone to falling asleep when lying down and relaxing, you might want to perform self-treatments while sitting up.

One of the beauties of Reiki energy is that when you perform a session on yourself, or even on someone else, you are drawing

Reiki energy from the universe. You are not expending any of your personal energy, so after a session you should not feel physically depleted or exhausted. If you were tired before performing a self-treatment session, you may in fact feel more awake and alert when the session is complete.

That is another benefit of self-treatment sessions, if you need a boost after work to get through your evening activities, doing a self-treatment session can provide you with that energetic pick-me up you might need.

As has been touched on a few times, the best healing comes from within. This means that you are the most instrumental source of your own healing. Self-treatment sessions give you the power to pursue that internal healing process. Even when you get Reiki healing sessions from another practitioner, you are still going to have to look within for the sources of imbalances and for the proper way to shift your energy and prevent future imbalances.

When performing self-treatment sessions with Reiki your intuition is going to be much more aligned with what is happening inside your own body. Therefore, you can get to the root of your imbalance faster and discover what will work for you in fixing it.

The body has such an amazing ability to heal itself. Unfortunately, modern societies impose limitations, jobs, and other restrictions that tend to work against the body's natural ability to heal itself. By aligning your personal energy flow and changing your energetic vibration, you are giving your body the means to heal itself. This healing happens on a physical, emotional, and spiritual level.

Reiki is a holistic healing energy. That means it heals all, it heals and balances on all levels of all the components of the body. Treating yourself with Reiki energy every day is going to keep your body in that alignment, so that you can focus more on your desires and goals in life and not sicken yourself with worry, stress, or be bogged down by physical pain.

Self-treatment sessions are great because of the flexibility in time and schedule that they offer you. Self-treatment sessions give you more control over hand positions and what is done in a session, or what Reiki symbols are used, if you've been attuned to Reiki symbols. Self-treatment sessions allow you to heal yourself from within, which is the most profound way to heal yourself.

Healing Crisis

Sometimes when going through the process of self-healing and shifting your own vibration, you can encounter what is called a Healing Crisis.

A healing crisis occurs when you begin a new course of study, or treatment, or pursue a new field of education, such as Reiki, and things don't seem to go as 'planned.'

An example could be that you experience chronic inflammation. This inflammation starts due to a single stressor to the body which results in a defensive response i.e.

inflammation. This stressor can be physical, emotional, external, or internal.

If the stressor is not identified and you continue to use the substance, practice the action, or follow the belief that triggered the inflammation, then the problem is just going to get worse. Your defense reaction will happen again and again, building on that inflammation until it becomes chronic.

Let's say that before you were dealing with the inflammation your body, mind, and spirit were operating at a level of 7 or 8 on a scale of 1 to 10, on most days. Now that the inflammation has become chronic, perhaps you are functioning more at a 4 or a 5 on a scale of 1 to 10 every day. You begin to adjust and learn to live with that chronic condition because it just becomes a part of you.

Suddenly, change can take place. It has been recommended that you try a new vitamin, that you talk to a new therapist, or that you look into a new course of study. You decide to give it a go. Initially, you might not feel any change and you could assume that it just didn't work. In some cases, you might find that you feel worse and you attribute the worsening feelings to the new method you tried.

This type of healing crisis is a common problem. What happens is, as the body, mind, and spirit are exploring something new or learning something new, it causes you to take a step back. The intention of the step back is to adjust your perception or perspective. This can sometimes happen when going through Reiki sessions and treatments.

It is important to remember that Reiki is not a heal all, nor it is an instant cure or fix. Reiki energy takes time to work. Additionally, it takes time to understand what needs to be shifted and changed to work towards a healthier lifestyle. Often times, if something doesn't work right away, people give up on it. That is why Reiki self-treatment sessions become so important!

Through treating yourself you can help your mind shift perspectives so that you truly get what you need from the path you are on. Self-treatments on a daily basis can result in more noticeable changes in your day to day life. This is why it is recommended that you document shifts and changes, no matter how subtle.

When you embark on a journey to heal yourself and strive towards a successful, fulfilled existence, a lot can happen. Emotions and traumas can be released, the work can seem slow and fruitless, but truly making a change in yourself isn't going to be easy or quick.

Some things to remember if you feel that you are experiencing a healing crisis are to:

Be Gentle with Yourself

Meditate

Hydrate

Breathe

Surrender

Perform Self-Treatments

Receiving Reiki from another Practitioner

There are many reasons to receive a Reiki session from an experienced practitioner. One of the major reasons to see a practitioner is because you feel blocked. This doesn't mean that you have an energy block, it means that you physically feel blocked in whatever you are experiencing and you are completely unable to help yourself.

Even with all the tools of Reiki self-treatments, crystal healing, and healing the chakras, you might encounter some traumas that cannot be resolved without a little help. If this happens, seeing a Reiki practitioner for sessions is a great way to help you move past that block enough so that you can start healing yourself. In this case, having a Reiki practitioner work on you is going to jump start your ability to work on yourself.

You may need to go for several sessions, or find that you want to continue seeing your Reiki practitioner as you work on yourself as well.

Other reasons to see another Reiki practitioner can be about experience and technique. You can learn a lot about Reiki by receiving sessions from another practitioner. You can learn new techniques and also discover new methods of applying Reiki. Everyone has differing experience levels and a lot of Reiki practitioners learn multiple energetic disciplines that you might find interesting.

Another reason to have a Reiki practitioner is for a sense of community. There are a lot of Reiki communities in local settings now. Joining a Reiki community is a great way to meet like minded people, share techniques and knowledge, and some Reiki communities trade free sessions when they meet.

This is just the beginning, you are going to keep learning and growing, so having other Reiki practitioners that can offer guidance and wisdom is such an asset.

Even if you become a Reiki Master, it is still recommended that you get Reiki sessions from other Reiki practitioners. The frequency of this is going to be a personal choice, however you shouldn't replace your self-treatment sessions with sessions from another practitioner.

It isn't uncommon for practitioners to have multiple other practitioners that they see for sessions. If you recall, after the 1980s, it was encouraged for Reiki students to study under different masters and receive Reiki sessions from different practitioners. Not only you can learn from them, but they can learn from you as well. It becomes an exchange of knowledge and growth for the both of you.

When looking for Reiki practitioners in your area, you'll want to find ones that you feel a connection to, that you resonate with. You might decide that you want to have some in-person practitioners, but then also have a Reiki practitioner that performs distance healing sessions. This continues to expand your Reiki network and your healing opportunities. Sometimes your intuition will guide you to a practitioner for a specific reason, but lead you to a different practitioner for another reason.

Many Reiki practitioners refine themselves to a specialty or a niche. For example, some practitioners will work only with clients who experience chronic pain. Others will work with clients specifically on healing past life and generational traumas. Other practitioners might focus on clients with mental illness such as depression or anxiety disorders.

There are many different reasons to get a healing session from someone else, and one of the most important reasons is because it feels good and is very beneficial.

Performing Reiki Sessions on Other People
When you perform a Reiki session on someone else, two things happen. The first is that you provide a widely beneficial healing service to a recipient who is in need. The second thing that happens is when you channel the Reiki energy through yourself you retain Reiki benefits for yourself, even if your focus is on your client. Definitely a win-win situation.

When performing Reiki on others, it is important to get their permission. That may sound obvious, but if you get attuned to Reiki Level II and have the ability to perform distance sessions, you won't need a client on your table to provide healing services. That being said, you always want permission from a recipient before performing a session. Without permission, you could unintentionally push someone into processing emotions they aren't ready to process which can have negative results.

Performing Reiki sessions on someone else has benefits for you that go beyond just channeling Reiki energy through yourself. Since Reiki is channeled energy through you, performing Reiki sessions on others won't drain you of energy. You shouldn't be putting your personal energy into a Reiki session, it should all come from the channeling of universal energy. When you act as the conduit for Reiki energy, you are a one-way conduit. That means as energy shifts and releases from your client, it can't travel back through the conduit into your body. Many other energy healing methods don't have that built in safety feature, so practitioners can inadvertently pickup energies that are released from the recipients. Reiki has not such risk.

Another benefit to performing Reiki sessions on other people is in the learning.

By working on others, your intuition can lead you to different hand positions and techniques that you might not discover while working on yourself only. Additionally, since clients and recipients will have different reasons for healing than you, your knowledge and understanding of energy and root causes of imbalances is going to expand and grow.

Having that wisdom will only help you as you progress on your own healing path. The point of self-healing isn't just to improve your physical, emotional, and spiritual health, but to allow you to grow and change with the knowledge and wisdom that you gain. Performing Reiki sessions on other people gives you the opportunity for literal hands on learning experiences.

Sometimes it takes working on another person to experience visions and sensations related to energetic shifts in the body. While working on yourself you can often feel the shifts occurring in your body, if you feel them in someone else, it takes your understanding of Reiki to a much deeper level.

Most practitioners who decide to provide Reiki healing services professionally to clients will rise up to at least Reiki Level II. It isn't necessary; however, it is recommended. If you don't want to offer professional services, you can still use the knowledge from Reiki Level I to offer complimentary healing services to friends and family or in a Reiki community.

Chapter 17: Reiki And Alternative Therapeutic Disciplines

With all of your new knowledge about the chakras and auras, you can understand more of what some of the other energy healing modalities are and how they work in relationship to your vibrational frequency. The chakras and auras as you now know are always being influenced by our activities, experiences, and mental states. You can shift your vibrational frequency with Reiki treatments, and you can also use some of the following applications to help you align, rebalance, purge, cleanse, and heal your chakras and auras.

Yoga

Most people in the modern world have heard of yoga, but if you have been living on a deserted island for the past several years, then allow me to explain the concept of yoga. Yoga is a series of postures or poses, combined with breathing styles and exercises, mantras, and meditations, to help the body, mind, and spirit center, ground, and attain wholeness.

The philosophy of yoga comes from the same ancient Hindu texts knows as the Vedas that the original theories about the chakras were written in. Yoga was already being established before Buddha was even born, and before Reiki was created by Usui in Japan in the early 20th century. The principles are largely based around the concept of healing the energy centers of the body to create a life of balance, humility, wisdom, and enlightenment.

There are several different styles of yoga that have different purposes, approaches, and outcomes and are mainly performed with the help of an instructor, either through online resources or in yoga studios. There is a public practice of yoga at this time that extends beyond the original Eastern borders from where it originated, demonstrating a global need for this kind of physical, mental, and spiritual practice.

Yogis, as they are often called, spend their whole lives living by the sacred practices that were originally written about so many centuries ago, dedicating their lives to the creative flow of personal life force to stimulate awareness and Universal consciousness.

There are millions of people practicing yoga today and there is a good reason for it: yoga stimulates the healing and release of stagnating, negative, and low vibrational energy to allow for a higher frequency on all levels. You can incorporate any kind of yoga practice into your Reiki healing schedule so that you are resolving the issues and blockages in more than one way.

Yoga studios are easy to come by in any community, or you can use online instructions and guided classes as a way to introduce you to the postures and breathing exercises before you advance to higher levels of practice.

Meditation

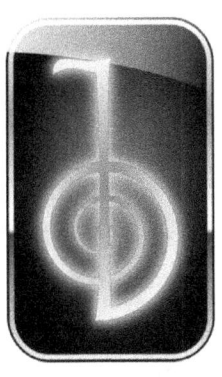

Meditation can certainly be a part of yoga, but you can also appreciate meditation on its own. Many people today are using meditation as a process to enhance their life skills and personal quality of life. It doesn't take much and as little as five minutes a day can be enough to change your frequency for hours.

There are a lot of us who need a few minutes of calm and repose between activities, at the end of a long, hard day, or as a way to kick start the morning. Meditation is an act of thoroughly connecting with the self and engaging in a moment of self-reflection. You may not think that this could have a long-term effect on you but it has actually been studied by doctors, therapists, and scientists to completely change your state of mind, emotions, and physical well-being.

An attitude of inward reflection helps you to slow your mind and engage with what you are really trying to tell yourself. It has a way of aligning you better with your higher mind, intuition, and positive attitude towards yourself and others.

Meditation lowers stress, relieves anxiety, dissolves depression, and quells fears and doubts. The practice of meditation is quite simple and all it takes is a few minutes of your time in an uninterrupted setting. You can sit, stand or lie down and you can take as little or as long as you need. Try five minutes at least, though, because anything less won't create much energetic change for your well-being.

When you meditate you are honoring your energy, collecting your thoughts, acknowledging your concerns, worries, and place in the world, as well as helping yourself align with a more powerful vibration that you can carry through your day.

With Reiki and meditation combined, you can help yourself create more awareness about your healing experiences as you maintain balance throughout the journey. Reiki healing treatments can cause some upheaval as old and outworn thought patterns, behaviors, emotions, and wounds come to the surface for healing. Meditation can assist the path you have to take to effectively heal these energies as you go.

Acupuncture

Acupuncture is an alternative healing practice that originates from the ancient methods of traditional Chinese medicine. The concept of acupuncture relates to using very small needles to prick the skin at specific points on the body. These points are described as part of the meridians of the body and where the Chi (life-force energy flows). Similar to the concepts of chakras and auras, Chinese medicine describes our vibrational frequency as Chi and considers it to flow through the body through channels called meridians. Each acupuncture point is thought to be a tiny energy center, like a chakra, that can become blocked and unhealthy.

The acupuncture needles are what alter the flow of the energy through the body and clear the channels so that your whole system can renew its balance and physical integrity. With all of the studies and research surrounding the benefits and results of acupuncture, it's amazing that there aren't more Western medical institutions employing this healing practice. It has helped people overcome addictions, stimulates regeneration of cells, heals the wounds created by chemotherapy, helps people with a variety of cellular disorders and dysfunctions, reduces stress, anxiety, and inflammatory conditions of the joints and body, and so much more.

Reiki and acupuncture both work to create healing within the energy systems of the body and can combine to create an effective unit of powerful healing force. Although Reiki uses a different system and method for clearing the energy of your chakra and aura systems, acupuncture needles are supportive of the same life-force field of energy within each person.

Crystals

What are crystals? You have probably held on in your hand, or at least seen one hanging from a chandelier, or in a New Age shop. Many people have associated crystals with pseudoscience healing methods that have no significant purpose other looking nice and chalk them up to being the baubles of the New Age community. They couldn't be more mistaken.

Crystals are actually high vibrational objects that emit frequencies more powerful than some people realize. The first microphones and gramophone needles were actually made with clear Quartz crystal because of its ability to conduct electrical currents and transform energy from one form to another.

If a Quartz crystal can create an amplification of sound and transform energy, what else can it do? Crystals and stones are capable of healing and transforming energy, just as Reiki and the other healing modalities you have learned about can. The crystals are mineral and elemental composites that are formed slowly over time in the Earth. Many of them come from specific places on Earth, while others are actually the byproduct of meteor showers and other direct contacts from cosmic rocks and debris.

A lot of crystals and gemstones are mined while others can be easily harvested from riverbeds, mountain paths, and other exciting outdoor landscapes. You can probably find a majority of the world's crystal and gem varieties at a local shop that specializes in them, and these days they are easy to purchase from online stores.

Crystals, like our chakras and auras, carry a frequency. Everything in the Universe has vibrational frequency and we just so happen to know that crystals work well with our energies because they are higher in frequency than most other objects. Quartz crystal has one of the highest frequencies and has been known to be effective in the healing of some diseases and cancers, as well as a tool to create spiritual awakening.

You can buy them or find them on your own, but either way, to cut it, crystals are a powerful natural element that has the energy you need to heal. You can lay them over any of your chakras and meditate with them to help you find a new balance and vibration. You can incorporate them into your Reiki healing treatments so seamlessly and they will only enhance the healing power of the Reiki experience.

As you get more and more acquainted with all of these tools for healing your vibrational frequency, keep in mind that they can all be beneficial to you on their own, but if you were to explore each of them through your healing practice, you would experience exponential healing and growth. Reiki is not limiting and invites anything that will help you heal your energy. After all, Reiki is Universal and opens you up to appreciating more of what these alternative healing methods have to offer.

You always have these resources to guide you on your path to self-healing and the choice is yours for how you choose to bring them into your life. Reiki can be a wonderful way for you to explore these alternative healing therapies and give yourself all of the support that you need right now.

In the next chapter, you will learn some of the tools to help you heal yourself with Reiki. If you are already attuned to Reiki energy by a Master, you may find these tools and techniques easier. If not, don't worry: you can still practice and learn your own way of introducing yourself to Universal life-force flow and channeling.

Prepare yourself to learn some new ways to approach healing and enjoy the ride!

Chapter 18: Black Tourmaline And Reiki

Black Tourmaline- One of my very favorite crystal. I have Black Tourmaline stones, a bracelet, a pocket stone and 3 pendants☐. It definitely shows my craze towards this stone. I have placed stones in each room, one under my wish and pendants for family. Kids are actually addicted to Black Tourmaline, they miss their pendant when I put the pendants out during full moon.

Every crystal lover knows that Black Tourmaline is the MUST HAVE stone for its powerful healing properties. Reiki and Crystals both have their own amazing healing energies and when both powerful healing energies combine, the outcome becomes double beneficial. The first and foremost thing to do is cleanse the crystal and infuse it with Reiki energy. We all know that crystals works with or without Reiki but crystals infused with Reiki makes the healing quicker, stronger and more powerful.

Black Tourmaline is a stone of protection. It is also called as Guarding Stone. Infusing Reiki to Black Tourmaline increases its vibrations to release negativity and blockages and gives powerful shielding and grounding.

Black Tourmaline as Protecting Stone- (Do not forget to infuse with

Reiki to double the benefits of the stone)

• Wearing or carrying this stone shields you from psychic attacks and psychic vampires.

• Shields you from negative vibes

• When Black Tourmaline is placed in home or work area, it provides protective shield around you and your home space or work space.

• Transmutes all negative energy to positive.

• Shields you from your own negative thoughts and fear.

• Stops these psychic vampires to suck off your energy; they won't be able to get a drop of your energy is Black Tourmaline is around your auric field.

- Wear a Black Tourmaline or place it in your wallet, purse, bag, and pocket, under your pillow, add in your bath or anywhere in your room.

Place is beside electronic equipment. Make an elixir of this stone and spray on self or space. Just keep this stone close to your auric field.

- Rubbing Black Tourmaline also brings good luck and happiness.

Black Tourmaline as Healing and Grounding stone-

- We all know how important grounding is for Reiki practitioners. Wearing or carrying Black Tourmaline makes you feel grounded and safe.
- Many times practitioner forgets to ground themselves before healing a client. Always make a habit to wear or put Black Tourmaline near the healing space to protect you and ground you.
- Black Tourmaline is directly connected to root chakra hence it helps balancing root chakra. It also connects us to Mother Earth.
- Helps reducing stress and addiction

- Place a Black Tourmaline on your Solar-Plexus and give Reiki to bring clarity and power.
- Meditating with Black Tourmaline brings more light to cells.
- Stimulates balance between left and right side of the brain.
- Also helps balancing work-and-play, pain-and-ease and high-and-low vibrations.
- Many times after giving healing, practitioners feel drain-out as they have absorbed client's energy. In that case, just hold Black Tourmaline in your palm and relax for a while. It deflects all unwanted energies absorbed from the client.

Black Tourmaline to absorb Electromagnet Energy-

- We are all the around electronic equipment and devices and accumulating electromagnet energy. Black Tourmaline helps absorb electromagnet energy.
- Give Reiki to the stone with the intention that it absorbs all electromagnet energy.

Place the stone near equipments and devices that emits electromagnet energy.

Black Tourmaline as Manifesting Stone-

• Write your wish on a paper. Draw Reiki symbols and chant its names.

• Fold the paper and put it under Black Tourmaline.

That's it. As simple as that. Black tourmaline removes negativity attached to your wish and further shield it, hence quicker manifestation.

Black Tourmaline Grid-

Setting a grid with Black Tourmaline removes negativity off your wishes and hence makes healing and manifestation faster.

Alternatively you can place Reiki charged Black Tourmaline stones in all corners of the room if you feel people with negative energy keeps entering your room. This is best done at work place or office where many known or unknown people tend to enter. Black Tourmaline absorbs all the toxic and negative energies and provide a shield to your room.

So, if you don't have Black Tourmaline stone, go and order one NOW☐

Dolphin Reiki

Dolphin Reiki was created by Mark Scott. Dolphins are considered to be master healers. They are here to help us and guide us. Reiki is a life force energy; In Dolphin Reiki, life force energy comes directly from Dolphins.

Dolphins have the ability to communicate on a higher spiritual level. Dolphins helps accepting and releasing negative emotions. When we hold on to pain and negative emotions, we build up emotional and physical problems for us. You don't need to be in presence of a Dolphin to be healed by them. Some even consider Dolphins equal to Ascended Masters and Archangels. Dolphins are also called angels of the sea.

In Dolphin Reiki, energy is transferred to someone by simply laying your hands on them or by distant healing. Dolphin Reiki heals the person as a whole- body, emotion and soul. To activate Dolphin Reiki, simply state

"Dolphin Reiki" three times and say "Dolphins, I call upon you to be with me and help me heal _____ (person's name)". The person who is getting healed by Dolphin Reiki may feel joyful, playful and peaceful and may feel engulfed in loving energies. A healing session may last about 30 minutes. Dolphins know exactly where the healing should go- body, mind, emotion or soul. You can call upon Dolphins even when using other healing modalities.

A Dolphin Reiki practitioner can also heal through breathing along with hand placement or directly blowing on the affected area to be healed. Activate Dolphin Reiki, inhale through nose, state your intention in mind and blow on affected area or organ through mouth. A client may be asked to use their own breathing exercise by inhaling through nose, imagining affected area is healed by Dolphin, and exhale through mouth.

For **_self-healing_**, place your hand on heart chakra. Activate Dolphin Reiki by saying "Dolphin Reiki" three times with the intention that all negativity be removed and all disease be healed.

For ***distant healing***, use any distant healing method. Call upon Dolphin and connect to Dolphin Reiki stating "Dolphin, I ask you to bless _____ (person's name) with your presence during healing _____ issues. Send healing for 15-20 minutes.

For ***fear release***- Sit or lie down. Take few deep breaths. Activate Dolphin Reiki and wait for a minute. You may or may not feel some soft vibrations. Mentally say, "Dolphin, I ask you to remove all the fear buried deep within me across all lives". Let the energy flow for 15-20 minutes. Imagine your body is swept by sparkling pure white water, sweeping away all negativity, blockages and fears.

Chakra cleansing- Sit or lie down. Take few deep breaths. Activate Dolphin Reiki and wait for a minute. You may or may not feel some soft vibrations. Bring your attention to root chakra. Mentally say, "Dolphin, please remove all imbalanced energies, negative vibes, fears, dust and debris buried deep within my root chakra". Let the energy flow for 3-5 minutes. Imagine your body is swept by sparkling pure white water, unblocking and cleansing root chakra. Do the same procedure for all the chakras. You will feel joyful and refreshed after this session.

Benefits of Dolphin Reiki-

• Physical, mental, emotional and spiritual healing
• Greater self-love
• Greater self-acceptance
• Loving relationships
• Lesser fear
• Deep inner joy
• Peaceful mind
• Manifestation of your deepest desires and more…

For any of the above given method, you can merge other reiki symbols too.

Chapter 19: Reiki Basics

The basics of Reiki will be taught in your first-degree training and as you get higher in degrees and levels of Reiju (attunement) you will learn more about the gifts of Reiki and how to practice it well. The elements of Reiki come together to promote a way of life and a belief that will help you stay grounded in the right energy and platform of healing to help you on your path of healing yourself and other people.

The pillars and principles of Reiki are from Dr. Usui's original format for teaching Reiki and will demonstrate the basic mentality of what Reiki embodies and helps to connect you to in your practice. You will also learn about what are called the Five Reiki Elements, although these were not originally taught by Usui and are from an adapted form of Reiki. You will learn about it here as many Reiki Masters have started to teach these elemental concepts and so you may find a Master who would like to train you with these kinds of techniques.

All of the basics of Reiki, together with what you have already learned about energy and how Reiki works, will help you find the attitude, respect, focus and admiration you need for the Reiki healing process. As you read, ask yourself what part of these principles you are already working with in your life and how you can improve upon them.

The Five Reiki Principles

Reiki is meant to be thought of as a healing practice. It may have been born out of a world religion, but it is not a religious practice. There are basic principles of Reiki that are meant to help you receive Reiki through an open consciousness and purity of intention and spirit.

The five principles were created by Usui and are seen here in these pages. They have gone through many alterations and additions, but this is as close to the original concept as you can get. These principles are useful to memorize so that you can implement them into your practice sessions as you prepare to work with a client. They serve as helpful reminders to keep you focused and in an attitude of healing and working as a channel of light and love.

They are as follows:

Today, I will not worry.

Today, I will not be angry.

Today, I will do my work with honesty.

Today, I will give thanks for all of my blessings.

Today, I will be kind to all living things.

These principles are simple and effective and are mantra for healing and growth. These five principles are what set you on the right path of healing and having an open heart to allowing Reiki to flow through you effectively for healing purposes. These affirmations, or mantras, are part of the basics of how your entire energy and life-force is able to accept Reiki and allow it to become a part of your every day life. It is a good practice to state these principles to yourself every day.

In Usui's clinic, he trained his students to meditate every morning and night on these principles. Your Reiki Master will likely not ask you to do this, but you may find that you will want to keep them handy in your mind for your healing practice and therapeutic work.

The Three Pillars of Reiki

The Reiki pillars give form to the principles and you could say that the principles are the foundation of the structure, and the pillars are what hold it up well. The pillars are actually just simple prayer poses, or meditations that help you maintain the principles within your practice. They are simple and effective and will give you the balance and energetic opening you need to ask for Reiki to help promote healing in the self and others.

The First Pillar: Gassho *(gash-show)*

Meaning: Two Hands Coming Together

This is a prayer position. It is the palms touching together and held out in front of the body at heart level, or if you are performing this hand position in a less formal way, the hands are up against the heart pointed toward the chin. A more formal gesture is seen with the palms together and the fingertips pointing out at a 45-degree angle, as a sign of reverence for what is in front of you or outside of you.

Either one of these positions is considered a Gassho and is used for prayer, meditation, a sign of respect, and so forth. The term "Namaste" is actually part of a Gassho and is used in a similar fashion, stating the word along with the hand sign means "I respect you."

A Gassho is often performed in a Reiki session as part of your greeting with a client and can be used throughout the session, or as you open and close your healing work with yourself, your client, and the Reiki energy flowing through you.

The Second Pillar: Reiji-Ho *(ray-zhjee-ho)*
Meaning: (Reiji) Indication of Reiki Power / (Ho) Methods

This is a three-step meditation, or prayer, to connect you to Reiki to allow you to be guided by the energy rather than just using hand positions. Additionally, this pillar is useful in distance healing practices.

First, you close your eyes and place your hands in Gassho and ask Reiki to flow through you, repeating the request 3 times (you can ask in your mind). Allow the Reiki to surge through you.

Second, you bring your hands in Gassho up to your third eye and ask for the health and recovery of your client on any and all levels, if it is needed. Here, you invite Reiki to go where it needs to go for healing. Ask Reiki to guide you and show you the way.

Third, Let Reiki pull you where you need to go and let go of the attachments you might have to controlling it. If you are not feeling like you are able to let the Reiki flow and guide you, you can repeat Reiji-Ho again, or simply use the hand positions over the chakras to help you direct Reiki into your client. When you are being guided, allow Reiki to do the work until you feel like you are no longer needing to work in any areas and then stop, as you are guided to do so.

Finally, perform another Gassho of gratitude and respect for the experience.

The Third Pillar: Chiryo *(chee-rye-o)*

<u>Meaning</u>: Treatment

According the rituals of this pillar, the practitioner will place the dominant head on, or above the crown chakra of the client being worked on (note: you don't have to physically touch a person in order to heal them with Reiki). From this position of rest over the crown chakra, the practitioner will wait for the inspiration, or impulse, to move in a direction.

Similar to Reiji-Ho, you are allowing the Reiki to guide you on your healing path with the person you are treating and when you perform this action, you are giving heed to the energetic "knowing" of the client (crown chakra) of where to go to treat them. Give free reigns to your hands and they will find the source of the pain, block, discomfort and place of treatment. You will remain in the places you are pulled to until you are released, as this will be when the pain is also released. Your hands will then move to the next place of treatment.

This pillar comes with more practice and experience in most cases, but is accessible to anyone who is open to working with Reiki. It tends to be a more direct healing treatment method, as opposed to the Reiji-Ho, which will have more flow overall. Chiryo will be more focused and slow moving.

These pillars are a part of the basic foundation and will give form to the structure of the principles you learned in the previous section. Practice these pillars along with the principles and you are well on your way to opening yourself as a channel of light and love.

The Five Reiki Elements

The Five Reiki Elements, as mentioned in the beginning of this chapter, are not a part of the original doctrine and teachings of Dr. Usui, however more and more Masters are teaching these practices to inform a more well-rounded position of energetic properties and healing practices.

The Five Elements are part of Chinese healing practices and are promoted in the Traditional Chinese Medicine techniques and Taoist philosophies. Wu Xing is another name for these elements together and they are earth, fire, water, wood and metal.

The reality of utilizing any element to understand the basics of Reiki is that it can show you another level of healing properties and practices in a fundamental and Universal way. In other cultural beliefs, there are the five elements described as being earth, air, fire, water and ether, or spirit. You can look at either of these platforms to help you study a deeper level of Universal truth to help you in your healing practices.

The elements are a practical approach to learning the lessons of what causes malnourishment, or health and healing, to the aspects of our whole selves. Every level of our being (mind, emotion, spirit, body) requires connection to these elements and with certain realities, too much or too little of one element can cause an excess or deficiency in another. It is similar to the chakra system and how an imbalance in one creates a need in another.

Interestingly enough, the chakras are each represented by an element, according to the traditions of their origin. (root=earth, sacral=water, solar plexus=fire, heart=air, throat=sound, third eye=light, crown=ether). Obviously, that adds up to more than five elements, but the perspective is that the basic elements are the basis of all life and all matter and so to understand the way the body, mind and spirit work, it is helpful to go over what the elements can be representative of in the healing process.

Since not all Reiki practices using these elements, you and the Master you study under, may have a certain approach to understanding and utilizing these elements. There are even entire books devoted to learning healing with this kind of approach and you can find more information through Traditional Chinese Medicine practices (Wu Xing) as well as in other off-shoots of the original Reiki practice laid out by Dr. Usui.

It is not a requirement of Reiki that you learn these elements, but it can be a very useful tool in your practice.

Other Practical Basics

There are a few other basics, some of which you have learned a little bit about in other chapters. These basics are all a part of what you might expect from a training experience and also how you can help yourself maintain good healing practices and structure.

Meditation and Techniques

Reiki is akin to a meditation. When you are working with a client to promote healing, you are in a deep trance of Reiki flow. It is like leaving your earthly self, long enough to transmit the direct flow of ULF into the energy centers of another. You can get better and better with time, and one way to help you remain focused in your treatment sessions is to practice meditation in general, before, and after your treatments. This can also help you relieve any of your own energetic issues or blockages so that you can stay grounded and open to assisting others in your work.

The pillars and principles you have learned are essentially meditations to practice Reiki and so if you are incorporating these principles into your work, then you are on the right path to staying grounded, centered and focused as a channel of light. The techniques you use in Reiki are also simple meditations that come with some practice and allowance of Reiki flow, so when you are practicing the pillars and the principles, you are effectively channeling Reiki. Other basic techniques that require a meditative mindset are the aura combing and energy assessment and other forms of assessment that utilize the third eye for "seeing" the problems and issues.

The technique of "energy sight" is highly common amongst Reiki practitioners and will begin to open up to you (if it isn't already) in your first-degree attunement when you begin to practice energy healing on yourself. You will often be able to see the auras, chakras, and what lies within them in a variety of ways. There really aren't any limitations to how these "issues" will present themselves when you are using the sight technique. You might see entire landscapes inside someone's energy field, or strange objects, creatures, or elements that need to be removed. It really just depends on each individual experience.

Practicing Reiki involves a lot of intuitive work and not just technique. You could say that opening yourself to channeling Reiki and using intuitive method is the main technique you will use to help you promote the healing process in another person. There are no practices that will help you better than following the flow of what Reiki shows you to do, and this is the powerful meditation of working with Reiki as a healing treatment.

Hands on Healing

As you have read in previous sections, hands on healing can be a basic part of your Reiki practice, although it is not necessary. There are basic hand positions that are options for you to use if you are not able to work in direct alignment with

Reiki guidance. Reiki guidance, as you now know, comes from practice and allowing the energy to pull and push you where you need to go. It feels almost like something else pushing your hands where they need to be to do the work. Your hands will even take on shapes and attitudes to help you pull or collect specifically shaped "pieces of energy" that need to be dragged out of the auric field.

The hand positions are incredibly simple tools assigned to certain placements and postures along the chakra system to show you where to work and where to let Reiki flow through. This process is not complicated and once learned will feel like a regular step-by-step approach to using Reiki healing techniques if you are not yet confident with letting Reiki chose where to go, as it asks you to follow along.

Mantras and Symbols

You will learn the specific Reiki symbols in another chapter, and they are considered one of the basics of a Reiki treatment session. You will not receive the symbols until your second-degree attunement and training, as this is the level that teaches you how to work on others, and not just the self. The symbols are just tools to direct and magnify, or enhance, the flow of Reiki and they can be very useful in other places as well, not just on a person. They can be incorporated into living and work spaces, in garden spaces and other environments.

Mantras are a part of the principles and pillars of Reiki and these can come up during any session. Also, as part of the symbol drawing technique, you will chant the name of the symbol, like a mantra, three times as you are drawing it. The mantra is stated in the mind and not allowed, in most cases.

Mantras and symbols are a powerful and effective tool, but are not always necessary. They provide more focused intention and as you get better acquainted with the general flow of a Reiki session, you may find that you only need one or two symbols every so often, while in other healing treatments you may need to use symbols and mantras often to promote a bigger energy shift and transformation in your client.

All of these Reiki basics are intended to help you see the overall platform of Reiki and how it is structured to help others and the self. All of these basics are part of the doctrine of Reiki and as Reiki transforms and is spread, new ways of approaching Reiki are permitted and accepted, as you have read with application of the five elements from another healing practice.

There are more ways than one to practice Reiki and this section only shows you the beginnings of what Reiki can do. In the next chapter, you will see some of the influences of Reiki and what some of the limitations can be in the process, as well as the benefits of this healing treatment.

Chapter 20: Using Crystals In Reiki

Since the beginning of time, crystals have been used to help people treat themselves or have been implemented by healers that sought to help others. Crystals have been associated with numerous healing and faith systems, and have featured prominently in all types of treatments all across the globe.

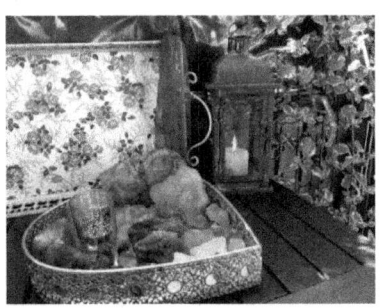

When it comes to the world of Reiki, crystals are used like a surgeon's tools—as precise and deliberate instruments for instigating positive change.

The initial, or foundational crystals that we will be looking at regarding Reiki are as follows:
- Rock Crystals
- Amethyst
- Fluorite
- Pink or Smoky Quartz

These crystals combine perfectly with the energy of Reiki, and also complement each other, as their qualities and capabilities differ yet span across the spectrum of usefulness, making them ultimately an all-encompassing combination of crystals.

Now let us examine the crystals in more detail, allowing us to understand both the crystals and their applications within Reiki.

Rock crystals

Rock crystals are perfectly transparent quartz. They have the most structured elemental building blocks in nature. Rock crystals are determined by their internal structure which is distinguished by both the qualities of perfection and balance.

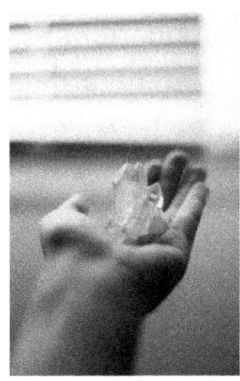

Rock crystals represents the highest stage of evolution in the kingdom of minerals and are quite universal in Reiki practice.

As a crystal, they are energetically neutral, meaning they can be used by anyone, and can also safely combine with other minerals.

Rock crystals are known to be able to stabilize the spiritual and physical strength of a person.

They can relieve pain, and have the ability to lower excessively high body temperature like fevers, etc.

Amazingly, this type of crystal never heats up. Rock crystals stay cool even when exposed to direct sunlight for extended periods of time.

This natural crystal is also capable of reducing bruising or head pain.

Rock crystals also have the power to improve the activity of the gallbladder, and they have a sedative or calming effect on the human body.

They can help with acute and chronic diseases of the liver and biliary tract too.

Rock crystals significantly contribute toward the correct functioning of the spinal cord and brain.

Rock crystals disinfect water. It can also be applied to wounds so that sun rays can filter through the stone and to the affected area, thus healing wounds. When passing through the crystal, ultraviolet rays kill bacteria, which contributes to a speedy cure.

Amethysts

The Amethyst is a crystal that helps to develop a person's inner abilities. It opens doors to higher spheres and stimulates an individual in such a way as to improve their capacity to comprehend universal wisdom.

It is also called the main stone of meditation. This is because it broadens the horizon of perception, promotes discernment and dynamically influences inspiration. To this end, the Amethyst is normally applied between the eyebrows.

The Amethyst has been proven to work well with high blood pressure, hyper-function of the endocrine glands, various inflammatory processes, psychological stress conditions, and insomnia.

A beautiful function of this crystal is that it calms the nervous system, which helps the practitioner/recipient to achieve peace, clarity and also significant strengthening of the memory.

Fluorite

Fluorite is a transparent or translucent stone. It can be found in various shades of color, such as colorless, blue, pink, yellow, green, purple, dark pink, black. Irregularity and varying intensity of the crystal, make it a very unique and elegant crystal.

In addition to having a pleasing appearance, Fluorite crystals are known to have the power to directly affect the energy centers (chakras) of the body, from the heart up to the crown. As a result, this crystal is able to remove the effects of stress, headaches, depression, anxiety, and emotional feelings. And considering the stressful situations that await most of us at nearly every turn in modern-day life, Fluorite truly is an invaluable tool by which to purify our minds and bodies from the toxic effects of our lives.

Fluorite also has a positive effect on the cardiovascular and nervous systems and the brain. The crystal is able to help with serious diseases such as epilepsy and multiple sclerosis.

Rose Quartz

Rose quartz is a healer of mental wounds, and are known within enlightened Reiki circles as the 'Stone of Emotional Health.' This wonderful crystal is invaluable because it helps us to feel the joy of life and love. This is achieved by applying the crystal to the heart area. The effect is a complete retuning of our spiritual focus. Often, our energy is divided, it is split between all the things that are happening in our lives. But by using Rose quartz on our heart area, our energy focus is shifted (radically and definitively) toward the direction of joy, and love. Providing instant fulfillment, and lasting peace.

The energy of this mineral helps us to adapt to, and ultimately make peace with and let go of, difficult life situations. It allows us to both surrender to the uncontrollable circumstances of life, while simultaneously bringing us into awareness and unison with our own personal power. It is a leveler of ego and a promoter of both the need to love ourselves, and to love those around us, regardless of their actions.

Conclusion

The subsequent stage is to quit perusing and to get beginning doing whatever it is that you have to do so as to guarantee that those you care about will be appropriately dealt with should the need emerge. On the off chance that you find that despite everything, you need assistance beginning you will probably have better outcomes by making a timetable that you plan to pursue including exacting cutoff times for different pieces of the errands just as the general consummation of your arrangements.

Studies demonstrate that mind-boggling undertakings that are separated into individual pieces, including singular cutoff times, have a lot more prominent shot of being finished when contrasted with something that has a general need of being finished yet no ongoing table for doing as such. Regardless of whether it appears to be senseless, feel free to set your own cutoff times for consummation, complete with pointers of progress and disappointment. After you have effectively finished the majority of your required arrangements you will be happy you did.

When you have completed your underlying arrangements for Reiki Self-Treatment, comprehend that they are only that, the lone piece of a bigger arrangement of readiness. Your best shots for general achievement will be stopped by setting aside the effort to learn whatever number fundamental aptitudes as could be allowed, which will be incorporated into our different books concerning the body's Chakra System. Just by utilizing your readied status as a springboard to the more noteworthy arrangement, will you have the option to really rest adequately realizing that you are set up for everything without exception that life chooses to toss at you?

www.ingramcontent.com/pod-product-compliance
Lightning Source LLC
Chambersburg PA
CBHW072008070526
44583CB00015B/1392